THE ALZHEIMER'S JOURNEY

It's Time To Get Organized

with

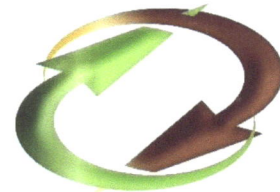

Personal Attache

Organizing Financial, Legal and Medical Records

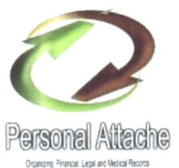

Personal Attache

Organizing Financial, Legal and Medical Records

Getting Organized Means

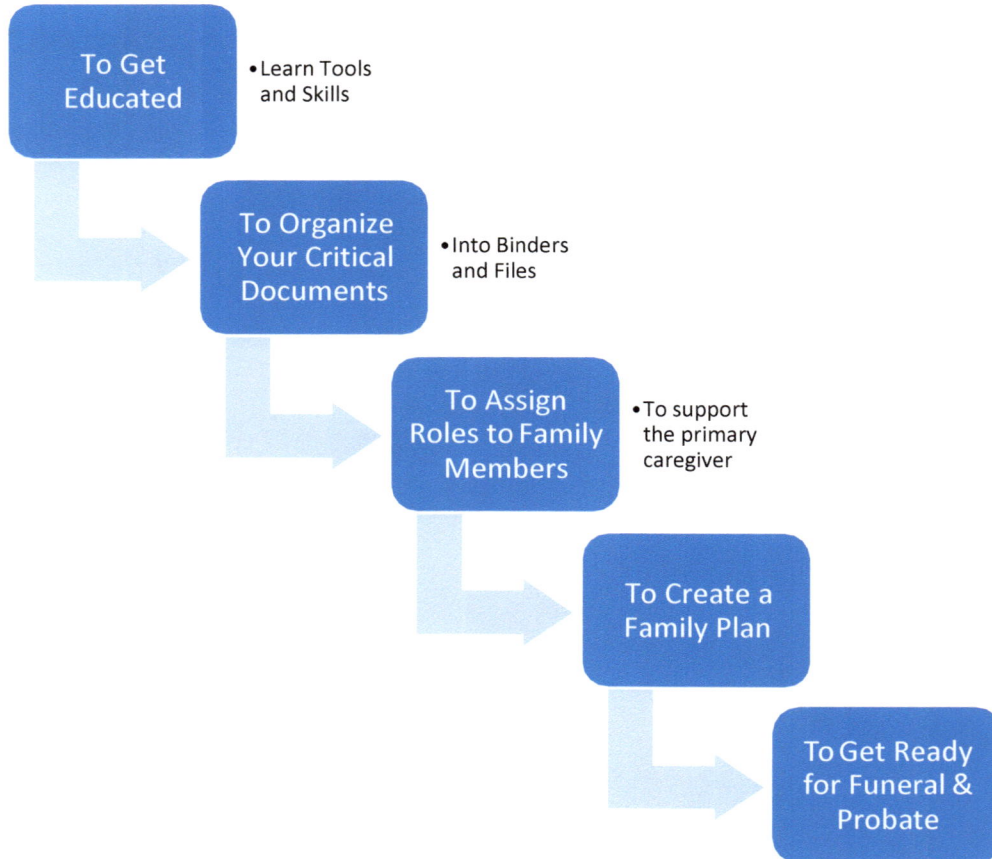

To Get Educated
- Learn Tools and Skills

To Organize Your Critical Documents
- Into Binders and Files

To Assign Roles to Family Members
- To support the primary caregiver

To Create a Family Plan

To Get Ready for Funeral & Probate

Personal Attache
Organizing Financial, Legal and Medical Records

FORWARD: Roy P. Poillon

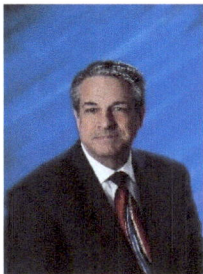

Mr. Roy Poillon has been serving the needs of Senior's in their home for over 25 years. His role was to design disease management in-home services for areas such as; COPD, Asthma, Diabetes, Wound Management and CHF. In order for these models to be successful it will require a family to be supportive and engaged in their loved one's care. In this work, he found that families are the nucleus and center for quality support in their loved one's disease management. However, at the same time he found that a family which is not organized, without direction or training, performs at a much less rate of success. It became evident; If the family doesn't get organized, then disease management support efforts are going to be for little gain. The family has to do its part, first.

Alzheimer's is a disease, and it too needs to be managed. This book is focused on getting the family organized to meet the challenges of their Alzheimer's disease journey.

Personal Attaché focuses on five key areas used towards getting the Alzheimer's family organized. 1. Organize the documents of their estate and home finance accounts, 2. Organizing the loved ones home medical records, 3. Organize the Legal Documents of their lives, 4. Organize for their life transition (Funeral Set-up), 5. Organize documents for Probate. This is difficult work and hopefully our study guide will make it a little easier to navigate through the maze of requirements. Therefore, to best serve your loved one "the whole family" needs to become involved in getting organized.

ABOUT US

The Alzheimer's Journey, It's Time to Get Organized, is our approach to get the family educated and empowered about managing the impact of Alzheimer's disease. To do this we created a center for learning. R~House Alzheimer's Family Learning Center. This is a multi-faceted organization that provides an Alzheimer's family with study guides, seminars, workbooks and on-line training webinars. But this will not be enough, so we have incorporated your local community, work place, church and social network. Mr. Poillon has four certifications in Alzheimer's disease from the Alzheimer's Association and had a personal experience with dementia. He is a 4th Degree Knight of Columbus and a member of the Marion Missionaries of Divine Mercy Association. This is his calling, and he sees it as God's love flowing through to your family. Getting your loved one organized is a matter of being compassionate it frees you up to practice your faith spirituality.

ABOUT YOU

Many families don't know where to begin when getting organized. They don't clearly see the "Roles and Responsibilities" that are needed for the Alzheimer's journey. To get organized, in a way that involves each family member; we need to assign roles and responsibilities, this will be the fastest most effective way for the family to move forward. In the family member's training we have included; Education on the disease, how to manage dementia behavior, identify the required areas that must be organized and ways to use faith practices within the Alzheimer's Journey. But, how ready and prepared are they to get involved and make a contribution? This is something each member must answer for themselves.

HOW TO USE THIS BOOK

In using this book, the reader should read it first, then come back and in the second reading complete each exercise and assignment. The assignments will build your knowledge in critical learning areas to strengthen the skills you will need in managing your loved one's care.

Prior to meeting as a family, it is best if each member has reviewed this book in order that they understand why certain steps are necessary.

R~house Alzheimer's Family Learning Center offers an On-Line Seminar which can be set-up by your family, to meet and review the development of their personal plan and activities in accordance with the sections in this study guide. Please contact us to set-up a date and time. Call: 440.385.7605 or email: www.wittsendconsulting.com.

Please know, you don't have to go through this alone. You have Witt's End Consulting, LLC to help.

 Respectfully,

R~House Alzheimer's Family Learning Center

Direct Line: (440) 385.7605
Email: wittsendconsulting@gmail.com

I. TABLE OF CONTENTS

Personal Attache
Organizing Financial, Legal and Medical Records

What It Cost to Be Disorganized

Getting organized in the area of finances — is one of the most important things we can work on, because these are things that add up fast and may result in lost money if not dealt with right away.

Getting Organized in Your Finances:

Some of these stress factors include:

- **Missed payments** - Most of your utility bills can be set up for automatic payment from a bank account. If you can't find the bill or miss payments, there will be finance charges and the possibility of being shut off from services.
- **Missed roll over dates** - Roll over dates on Certificates of Deposit (CD's) and other time sensitive investments can result in lost financial gains.
- **Missed opportunities** - Most financial opportunities are time sensitive. Knowing when to act and having the right documents in place is typically how to take advantage of these opportunities.
- **Emergency Responses** - When you need a document during an emergency and there are financial follow through tasks, it is now a matter of "now not later", that you will need to find these documents.
- **Overdraft protection fees** - By this we mean the transfer from your savings account to your checking account that happens when you overdraw the checking account but have the savings to cover it
- **Out of control spending** - When your loved one spends without good judgement do to Alzheimer's and you do not have a system to track this behavior.
- **Insurance policies** – You need the document in order to understand the policy and coverage of the insurance.

A lot happens when we cannot find things. The stress builds up, exhaustion and then mis- directed anger is the result. Take the time now, to give yourself a break later. Get organized by starting with your finances.

Getting Organized in Your Legal Affairs:

- Greater legal fees are paid by those who do not plan their affairs ahead of time. Also, by the time you need to use legal documents, this is typically not the best time to go searching for them or to find out you do not have them.

- There are many reasons why we put off doing our legal paper work and legal planning. It is time consuming, we don't know where to start and it is expensive. These are three reasons to do them now, while you have the time, while you can gradually learn what you need to know and can spread out the cost by putting the legal fees into your monthly budget. This legal work takes time, so start early.

- Planning ahead by getting the legal affairs of your loved one completed now is a good use of your time. It will greatly reduce your stress later.

Getting Organized in Your Healthcare Profile:

- In healthcare many doctors have what is called EMR (Electronic Medical Records). And that is good, but what if you are in a hospital ER and it is not your regular health network. They will not have that system's records; therefore, they will not have your loved one's records. In the Alzheimer's journey it is likely that your loved one will be seen by many different specialists. Keeping track of them in a Medical Records Binder will make that task a little easier.

- Also, Rehabilitation facilities, Respite stays and alternate site providers will not be on the health systems EMR network. Neither will your local pharmacy.

- Another area of why it's a good idea to have a Medical Records Binder is the labor of tracking all the appointments past present and future. Plus, if a family member needs to step in and take the loved one to an appointment, this binder will help to fill in some of the blanks. The binder allows others to help.

Introduction

Something Seems Wrong

In the start of Alzheimer's, there is a period of time when you are noticing that something just doesn't seem right about your loved one. Typically, a spouse, daughter or son will start to question themselves as to "Do I really see this or is it just me looking too close"? Your journey with this disease begins at the point of diagnosis. A timeline and progression of sorts has been identified with specific stages and known issues that will follow.

The family cannot go through the Alzheimer's journey alone. They will require extensive support during their loved ones decline. This support will come from four primary resources. Unfortunately, there is no one single resource structure that provides all four.

Each resource has its own structure. In many cases accessing these structures can be very challenging. The problem is many of these resources do not completely understand the needs of the Alzheimer's family. They are set up to provide services, but not necessarily for the exact needs of this type of family. Because of the support structures complexity, and their lack of understanding, it is best to use a model that can extract what the family needs from each resource.

4 Primary Support Structures:

1. **The Family Support Structure:** The family members are a resource support structure for the primary caregiver and loved one.

2. **The Church Support Structure:** The church is a resource support structure for the family members, primary caregiver and loved one.

3. **The Community Support Structure:** The community (professional services, medical, govt agencies and non for profits) is a support structure for the family members, primary caregiver and loved one.

4. **The Employer Support Structure:** The employer is a support structure for the primary caregiver.

The reason accessing the Four Primary Support Structures presents a problem is because they do not automatically show up at your front door. They offer services and leave it up to you to find them. In this two-part seminar the family will organize the critical documents and records so each of the 4 Primary Support Structures can be successfully navigated.

By using this organization model the family will approach each structure in a united, organized and proactive way to ensure the best outcome. In each section are "Assignments", you are expected to complete each assignment before continuing.

Getting Organized, Keeps Us on Our Path

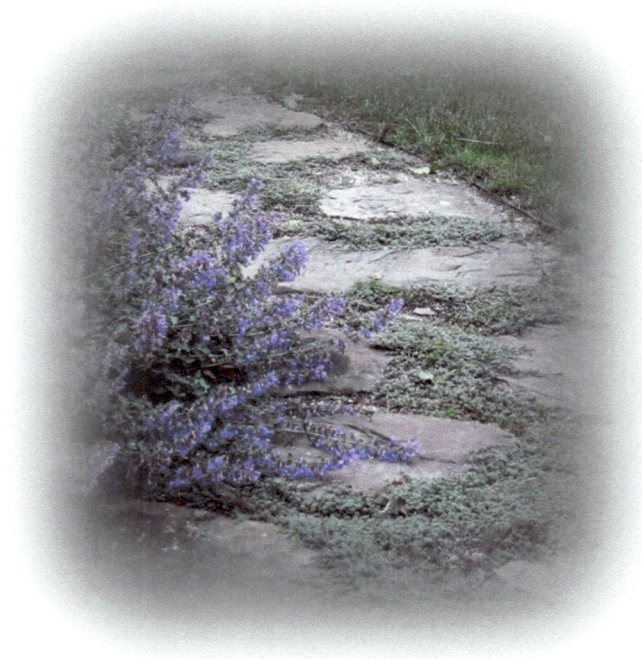

[40]But everything must be done decently and in order"

1 Corinthians 14:40

CHAPTER ONE

Getting an Assessment, Getting the Diagnosis

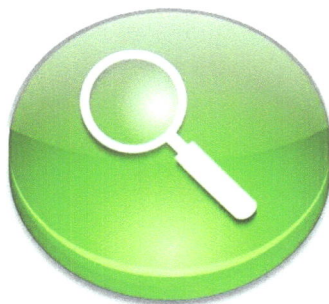

Getting an Assessment

An Alzheimer's Family Journal Entry:

There have been some occasions where our loved one is not acting the same and they seem to be displaying behavior that is significantly different from how they would normally act.

Therefore, we are going to use the 10 Signs of Dementia to see if this behavior matches up with the behavior that is identified on this list. (google: "10 Signs it's Alzheimer's")

Our conclusion was; the behaviors that we are observing are not an exact match to all that is on the list. However, there are enough criteria matches which warrants further review. We started looking for consistent behavior patterns to make sure it was not just a single event. We did see a pattern and for this reason we have scheduled an appointment with the "Brain Institute" for an assessment. We want a thorough exam and at the Brain Institute there is a multi-disciplinary team of Neurologist, Social Worker, Occupational Therapist and Psychologist that will perform this assessment. We feel this is a better approach than just a single doctor or primary care group practice.

In preparation for this visit we used the check list "getting ready to visit the doctor" www.alz.org/documents/national/ed_doc_checklist.pdf.

The family member who is most familiar with our loved one will attend the physician visit and be present during the assessment. Their attendance is required in order to provide historical information in an interview with the physicians team. They will also bring in a brown paper bag with all the pill bottles that our loved one is currently taking and a list of allergies that we know about.

Family Reflection:

This family is facing an unknown situation. They feel it warrants closer review. By getting an assessment in place of waiting, they can make better choices about care, plan for future needs and practice a higher quality of life care with their loved one.

Clinical Review:
Their loved one is now showing their brain cells are dying. This has been taking place for over the last 15 years. At this point the diminishment has gone far enough to where it is starting to show in the way their loved one is able to function regular brain driven skills. The disease is Alzheimer's, the behavior is dementia. This is when most families determine that what they are seeing is real.

Alzheimer's Family Spirituality:
Fear is heightened from what we do not understand. It can cause us not to move forward and avoid what we are not sure about. Because we cannot rationalize what is happening we need to rely on our faith. Our faith is in something that is greater than ourselves, stronger than ourselves, wiser than ourselves, so we lean on it to help us have courage in what is difficult to accept. We are reminded from our religious practice that there is Divine Mercy which we can receive through prayer and connect with through meditation. Here is where we need to ask for God's help to understand our journey and provide us with what we need by giving us His divine love, through His Mercy for us all.

Spiritual Consideration:
This can be a good place to gain a deeper understanding of the Lord's Divine Mercy. Through this meditation you will gain a stronger grasp of how Divine Mercy works in your life.

ASSIGNMENT:

View a Video:
Go to www.youtube.com, look up:
Early On-Set Alzheimer's disease: Jim's Story | OnMemory.ca

Read an Article:
www.Alz.org search Doctor's Visit Checklist

Reference the Alzheimer's Association Website:
http://www.alz.org/alzheimers_disease_10_signs_of_alzheimers

Go To:
www.formed.org see tab: Programs, See: Divine Mercy Self Retreat

Personal Attache
Organizing Financial, Legal and Medical Records

Getting the Diagnosis

An Alzheimer's Family Journal Entry:

At the physician's office we planned to have a lot of testing done, and then return several weeks later for the results. Ref: http://www.alz.org/alzheimers_disease_steps_to_diagnosis.asp

What we are looking for is a **primary diagnosis**. This diagnosis will be staged 1-7 and we will come back every 6 months (avg.) for a re-evaluation.

Family Reflection:

We went to this appointment with an understanding this is not an easy disease to diagnose. In fact they will likely eliminate all other possibilities in order to determine if it is Alzheimer's disease. This is because there are many diseases that create dementia, but 80% of dementia cases are Alzheimer's. The assessment will give us a primary and possibly a secondary diagnosis. We will use this diagnosed result as a dashboard to record and understand our loved one's current condition, then share it with the other family members. We understand this condition will progress in diminishment of the brain and therefore regular follow up visits will be required to gauge the progression of the disease.

ASSIGNMENT:

View a Video:
Getting the diagnosis:
https://www.youtube.com/watch?v=LieVEfI4luw

Reference the Alzheimer's Association Website for the stages of progression
www.alz.org/alzheimers_disease_stages_of_alzheimers.asp

Communicate results in a family meeting.

An Alzheimer's Family Journal Entry:

We need to inform the family about the diagnosis. The way that we do this is important. To just blast it out to everyone in the family is not a healthy way for this to be announced.

Announcing the diagnosis to the family, means that we are the barer of bad news, (does the term "don't kill the messenger" come to mind?). The best way for us to do this is in person (if possible).

Conversation with another family member: (Use this as your template)

- As you know we visited the Doctor and have received their results.

- The assessment was done using the most advanced methods of considering all the possible factors.

- These tests included neurology, psychology, occupational therapy and

  pharmacy They combined their findings, met on our case and their

  conclusion is: xxxx Here is what that means: xxxx

- Here are some of the broader details of what we can expect: xxxx

- They have strongly recommend that we handle this news together as a family so each person has the same information.

- This is hard news for me and you to face, but if we work together I know we can get through this.

- Our first steps is to look at the facts that surround this type of

  disease We will want to get educated and unify around

  supporting each other.

- We will want to learn about the best ways to handle our loved one so they get the best of what we are as a family. I believe that together we can give the most valuable gift, our time and support of each other during this journey.

- Because it last for a long period in time, we would benefit by creating a plan and taking roles to share the load of responsibilities.

o It is best, if the roles assigned are based on what each of us has as a certain skill set and is good at doing.

o Together, we will have to make a lot of important decisions. We need to understand that some of our decisions will not go as planned and we may not realize this until after they are done. So we can only do the best we can do, and need to accept that we tried with what we had at the time.

o We can expect many things will change and by trying to keep it all the same, it may make it more frustrating and stressful. So accepting change *"is required"* and could be a healthy approach. But we can keep the changes to only those that are needed and it is suggested that we wait to make a change, up to the time that the change is required.

o Here's the good news; there is a lot of quality and useful information out there for us to use. And there are people who will help us if we seek them out and bring them closer.

o Also, we have our spiritual faith which is something that a lot of people have told me is what got them through this journey. So, let's plan to include spirituality into our family's journey.

o The next step is to get everyone together in a room. We can meet at my house, what day of the week do you think will work best for you.

o Before you leave I have a sheet from this book I am reading, The Alzheimer's Journey, It's Time to Get Organized, and it has some "how to get started" tips.

o I would like for you to order this book and start reading it before we meet. That way we can begin our discussions from a point of an alike understanding, as to what we will experience. See (Appendix, An Alzheimer's Family Initial Meeting Agenda).

NOTE: *It is in the announcement of an Alzheimer's diagnosis that a family realizes things are going to change, significantly. Some will pull back from the announcement, "How could this have happened, could it have been avoided, maybe it will stop progressing or go away". This will be due to a lack of their education about the disease. I am sorry but none of these will apply to your situation. You did an assessment, you have a diagnosis, the faster you come to grips with this diagnosis, the better you will survive the journey. Our advice is to be understanding of the person pulling back, each will have to face this announcement in their own way. When it is presented, each person will have to travel their path, and determine for themselves how they will deal with this news.*

By getting through the shock of the diagnosis and into the education about the disease and how to handle the dementia related behavior, this will speed up the time it takes to come back to the family and be a valuable partner in the support team. So, education is your best next step. Please consider; you cannot rush them, they are on their own time line in dealing with this news. This is when you can show your family member compassion and understanding and that you will be there when they are ready.

Frequently Asked Questions: FAQ

1. **What should we be doing, now that we know it is Alzheimer's disease?**

You have already taken the first step, there was an assessment and there is a diagnosis. You are now becoming aware that life will be different for the next several years. To get educated about the disease, how it progresses, how to manage the dementia related behavior and getting your family affairs in order are some of the next steps.

2. **You Need to Get Educated?**

Don't Skip Over This.

Take the time, it's worth every minute.

ASSIGNMENT:

Go to www.hcinitatives.com and take their on-line training. View www.teepasnow.com youtube video's, all of them. Read every page on the www.alz.org site. Take the Alzheimer's training: www.alz.org/essentialz/

3. **Learn how to manage the Dementia Related Behavior?**

This disease comes in 7 stages, the first three are slow and mostly go un-noticed. The stage where most families will seek an assessment is the Early On-Set stage. Then to follow are the Mild Stage, Moderate Stage, Late Stage and End of Life Stage. A typical duration is 7-12 years.

In the above education tracks you will learn about what behavior presents in each stage and in what ways it worsens as the disease progresses. You can revisit this learning prior to each stage. This will prepare you for what will come next.

4. Get organized? Do this now, because later in the disease there will be no time.

You will organize the documents of our loved one into a file system that you will need to use. The handling of documents is performed by you, not them. The level of work is extensive, therefore, in this book we will have you assign workloads to your other family member by giving them "Roles & Responsibilities".

5. How can we plan to involve God?

Ask Him. Always be seeking "His Will" to be done in place of your will. And trust in Him completely. Pray the Divine Mercy chaplet at 3:00pm hour. Pray the rosary daily. Believe in His Mercy and love for us all. He is always with us, He never abandons us, He answers all prayers.

6. Are there known issues that we will have to face in this journey?

Fortunately Yes, we do know them. Many of the issues you will have to face as a family are known and can be planned for in your journey. This is done according to the stage you are in. Therefore, your family can plan in advance, get educated and be proactive. Although most issues will have to present their circumstances in order for the family to know exactly how to best respond, it is still a good idea to be prepared.

7. Is there a standard model for making good decisions?

Most families are not accustomed to making group decisions. So, by accepting a standard model now, this can be helpful later. In this book we suggest a standard model for family decision making. Use it in a way that best meets your family's specific needs and style. It allows everyone the chance to participate in the decision-making process and may bring the family closer together. When meeting as a family for making a decision, start with a prayer, ask for God's guidance before you begin.

What is the number one thing we need to keep in mind?

Your Family Values. The values that your family treasures above all other things in life. That is what you should use to guide your actions and decisions going forward. Ask first, what are our values? Then address the issue or question with this in mind. In this book is an exercise to determine as a family, what are your values.

Who needs to get organized?

ANS: *Organize the loved one's affairs first. Then organize yours.*

CHAPTER TWO:

Assess Your Current Situation

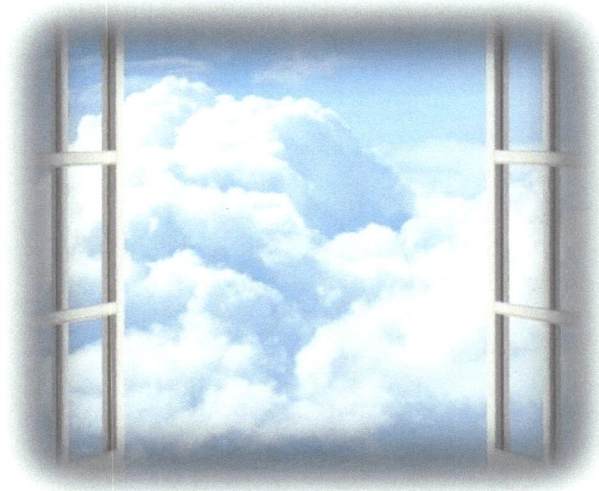

Assessing Your Current Situation

In this section your family will likely ask, what assets and documents are required to be organized? The answer may surprise you. Everything that is a document which reflects value to your loved one's life should be organized.

For many families where to get started may not be so obvious. Therefore, we have assembled an "Asset Evaluation Card" for your family to use in finding; what you have, what you do not have, and compare it to what you will need to have.

This sounds like fun, doesn't it? Well, not really, but taking an inventory of what you have is an essential step towards getting organized. Let's face it, if this were fun you would have already done it.

ASSIGNMENT:

Go through all of the known places where your loved one has documents filed or stored. Collect these items into one place. Separate them by category: Financial, Legal, Medical, Social and Spiritual. Then take an inventory of what you have been able to find.

By using the following *Asset Evaluation Card's,* you will record what you have, what you do not have, and from there you will more clearly see what you need to get.

Personal Attache
Organizing Financial, Legal and Medical Records

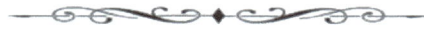

Financial Evaluation Card

In the area of Financial Assets, it is important to identify any and all financial assets as well as statement of debt, investments and insurances.

CATEGORY (Financial)	YES	NO	MAYBE	NOTES
Bank Account List				
Investment Account List				
Insurance(s) List				
Person Property Appraisals				
Auto Tile				
Real Estate Deed(s)				
Pension				
Social Security Payments				
Disability Payments				
Alimony Payments				
Business Partnerships Equity				

Personal Attache
Organizing Financial, Legal and Medical Records

Legal Evaluation Card

In the area of legal documents, it is equally important to identify what you do have from what you don't have and need to go get.

CATEGORY (Legal)	YES	NO	MAYBE	NOTES
POA Healthcare				
POA General				
Will				
Living Will				
Social Security Card				
Medicare Card				
Do Not Resuscitate (DNR)				
Commercial Business Partnerships				
Trust(s) Documents				
Promissory Notes				
Partnerships				
Guardianship Documents				
Letter to Loved Ones				

This is an area that may require cooperation from the staff at your physician's office. If you have multiple offices, it is important they all have the same basic information about your loved one.

CATEGORY (Medical)	YES	NO	MAYBE	NOTES
Health Plan Card				
HIPPA Release Form				
List of Medications				
List of Allergies				
Primary Diagnosis Report				
Previous Lab Results				
Documenting discussions with Physician				
Document Observations Log of parent condition				
Any Addictions, history or current				
Pharmacy Card				
List of non Pharmaceuticals				

Stress Indicators Evaluation Card

These are areas of the Primary Caregivers life that may influence their ability/capacity to cope with the demands of being alone in the role of primary caregiving. Nothing listed here would disqualify the person from being a successful primary caregiver. This is an awareness list that greater support will be helpful when considering their needs in this role.

CATEGORY (Caregiver)	YES	NO	MAYBE	NOTES
Attending a support group				
Regular Exercise				
Average Nutrition				
Spirituality Practice				
Working with sustainable income				
Completing Course work, academics or work				
Receiving Family Council Therapy				
Using Meditation				
Actively Participating Family Member(s)				
Involved Spouse				
Children at home				

Personal Attache
Organizing Financial, Legal and Medical Records

Support Network Evaluation Card

This card is used to determine the extent of the families support network. What is in place, set-up and established.

CATEGORY (Health Team)	YES	NO	MAYBE	NOTES
Active Primary Care Physician				
Neurologist team				
Psychiatrist				
Spiritual Minister				
Social Worker / Case Manager				
Occupational Therapist / Physical Therapist				
Home Health Aid				
Pharmacist on team				
Mail order disposable medical supply company				
Mail order Pharmacy				
Involved Spouse				
Regular Friends				
Any disabled dependents in the home				

Personal Attache
Organizing Financial, Legal and Medical Records

Guess What?

Your Asset Evaluation Cards are Completed !

Well not really or kind-of...

THE ASSET INVENTORY

At this time, you have taken an inventory and identified what Assets you **"do"** have. Now it becomes clearer as to what Assets you **"do not"** have, and what you likely **"still need to get"**. For this reason, the next step is to set-up a plan and collect the things you need, then place them all together into an organized binder. These binders can be organized by Asset Category.

Asset Category:

- ☐ Financial Binder
- ☐ Legal Binder
- ☐ Medical Records Binder
- ☐ Support Network Binder
- ☐ Spiritual Support Binder

Each binder can be assigned as a responsibility to a selected family member. That person will take up the role and responsibility of managing and updating their binder.

Role Assignments:

- ☐ Financial Person
- ☐ Legal Person
- ☐ Medical Records Person
- ☐ Support Network Person
- ☐ Spiritual Support Person

Assignment, Score your results:

SCORE your results. Go back through the last few pages of Asset Evaluation Cards and pick out what you don't have. Take the time to determine if that Asset applies to your family needs. If you will need it, then get it. Next, put "getting that asset" into a To-Do List and assign it.

By taking the Asset Inventory, and then SCORE it for follow up action, you will now have all the Asset documents you need to successfully move forward.

CRITICAL DOCUMENTS GO HERE

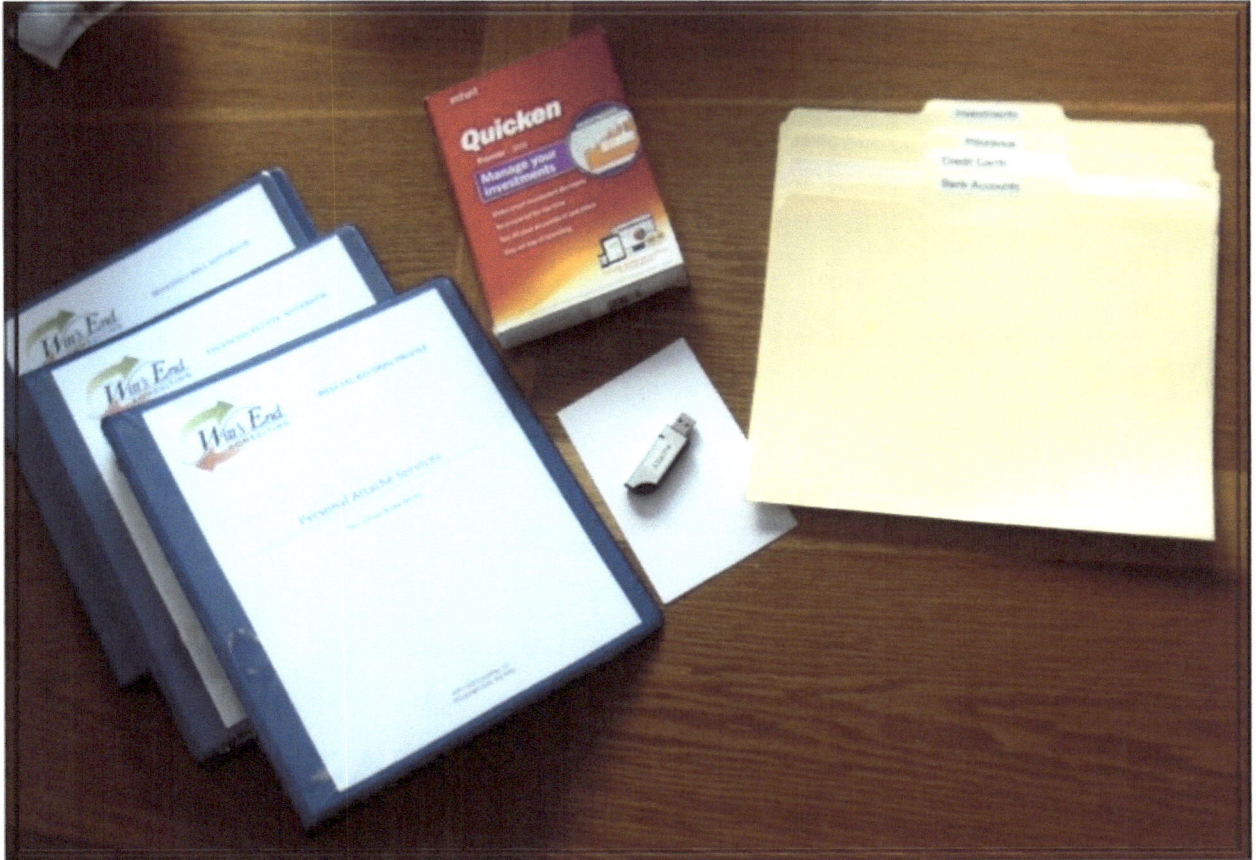

Office Max/Staples

- ½ inch binder
- ☐ Avery Tab Dividers
- ☐ Jump Drive
- ☐ Folders

Email wittsendconsulting@gmail.com and request the MS Word Documents for these templates.

CHAPTER THREE:

Assigning Family Members
Roles & Responsibilities

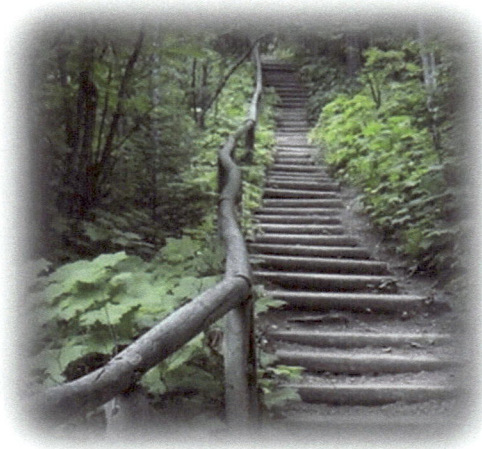

5 Each of you must take responsibility for doing the creative best you can with your own life. 6 Be very sure now, you who have been trained to a self-sufficient maturity, that you enter into a generous common life with those who have trained you, sharing all the good things that you have and experience. Galatians 5: 5-6

Assigning Roles and Responsibilities

First Step, Assign Family Member Roles

"Wives, submit to your husbands, as is fitting in the Lord. Husbands, love your wives and do not be harsh with them. Children, obey your parents in everything, for this pleases the Lord. Fathers, do not embitter your children, or they will become discouraged" (Col. 3:18–21).

God's plan has always been that inside a family, we are accountable to each other.

It is for this reason that we will take the time to allocate the work load of a primary caregiver to all those members of the family. Everyone has a role to play, in fact we have always had a role to play in our families, it was just rarely pointed out and written down on paper.

In this section, we will identify your roles and what area each of you will take as a responsibility to support the family.

Assigning Roles:

1. Who
2. Will Be Responsible to oversee What
3. How it will be done.
4. Determine what resources are needed.
5. When it will be completed
6. Report to family the progress.

The goal of assigning these roles and responsibilities is to take them off the role of the Primary Caregiver. At the same time, we use and apply the gifts and talents that are available from within each family structure. Everyone has a place to contribute and no one is left out.

"There are different kinds of spiritual gifts but the same Spirit, there are different forms of service but the same Lord, there are different workings, but the same God who produces all of them in everyone"

1 Corinthians 12-4

ROLE DESCRIPTION: The __Financial Role__ is alike one of a company Chief Financial Officer or Accountant. The affairs of the estate would be included to this role and also support of probate documents for timely court processing. Included to this list are monthly budgets and bills paying, managing financial investments and insurances as well as investment statements and bank account management. This person is not the final decision maker, but does contribute works that support the final decisions.

ROLES: _____

1. Tasks that involve all of the loved one's financial affairs.

2. Tasks that involve the loved one's real estate property.

3. Tasks that involve the loved one's possessions above a stated dollar amount.

4. Decision participation in affairs involving expenses, past and projected.

5. Monitoring and reporting the cost of living budget, medical bills (follow up) on payments.

6. Matters of Insurances.

7. Matters of debt collection responses and planning.

8. Matters of receivables in payments, interest, earnings, promissory notes, etc.

9. Matters of personal property

OTHER: _____

*ROLE DESCRIPTION: The <u>**Legal Secretary Role**</u> is one of coordinating the legal aspect of the loved one's estate and personal care, the completing and process filing of legal documents. They would participate in the preparation of documents for legal decisions, but not be the final decision maker.*

ROLE: _____

1. Tasks that involve the loved one's legal affairs.

2. Tasks that involve the loved ones legal responsibly for real estate Property.

3. Tasks that involve the loved one's legal possessions above a stated dollar amount.

4. Decision participation in affairs involving healthcare from a legal perspective,

5. Identifying all past and projected issues of the loved one and their legal accountabilities.

6. Monitoring and reporting the status of all legal affairs as it is related to their place of

   living, contracted services, medical bills, monthly bills and financial interest.

7. Matters of Insurances and investments from a legal perspective.

8. Matters of debt collection responses and planning from a legal perspective.

9. Matters of receivables in payments (what's owed to the loved one), interest, earning,

   promissory notes, etc. from a legal perspective.

10. Matters of personal property from a legal perspective

11. OTHER: _____

Personal Attache
Organizing Financial, Legal and Medical Records

*ROLE DESCRIPTION: The **Medical Records Organizer Role** is the one who organizes the medical records and health related documents for the loved one. They also assist in coordinating healthcare services and appointments.*

ROLES: _____

1. Tasks that involve the loved one's medical affairs documents, appointments and communication with alternate healthcare medical teams.
2. Tasks that involve the loved ones Medical Health Records.
3. Tasks that involve the loved one's appointment preparations.
4. Communicating and researching the facts for decision making: participation in affairs involving health and medical services. Knowing the labs, diagnosis test results, pharmacy drug interactions and side effects, allergies.
5. Monitoring and reporting the outcome of tests results and follow up to doctor's "plan of treatments". To do the research on these tests and communicate the facts.
6. Assist in getting to and from appointments.
7. Continuous Updating of the Medical Records Binder.
8. OTHER: _____

Let us remember that with God nothing is impossible; and as we read and hear his promises, let us turn them into prayers, Luke 1:38, *"I am the Lord's servant; let it be done unto me according to thy word".*

Personal Attache
Organizing Financial Legal and Medical Records

ROLE DESCRIPTION: The <u>Support Network Coordination Role</u> is alike one of a company Director Human Resources. The affairs of coordinating services, social outlets and family gatherings. This is a focus of creating balance, harmony and strong communication channels.

Roles: _____

1. Tasks that involve the loved one's support network from the community and family.

2. Tasks that involve the loved one's immediate family communication link, frequency and quality of life check-in's and acts of being compassionate.

3. Organizes family meetings or skype conference calls.

4. Tasks that involve follow-up's with the loved one's family siblings, associations, parish volunteers, etc.

5. Tasks that involve allowing the primary caregiver to participate in outside activities. Also, coordinating friends and support groups for the primary caregiver.

6. Home Health Aid and Respite services for the primary caregivers support.

7. Mail Order Medical Supply's and mail order pharmacy coordination.

8. House Cleaning Service

9. Address all Yard and House Maintenance issues.

10. Issues of safety in the home and home security.

11. Getting to and from appointments for both the loved one and the primary caregiver.

12. Making sure the primary care giver has time and space for personal exercise, grooming needs, and time away from the house each week.

13. OTHER: _____

Personal Attache
Organizing Financial, Legal and Medical Records

ROLE DESCRIPTION: The <u>Spirituality Coordinator Role</u> is one ensuring the spirituality needs of the loved one and primary caregiver are identified and being met with an adequate degree of support.

Roles: _____

1. Tasks that involve ensuring the loved one and primary caregiver receive communion (the eucharist) on a regular bases.

2. Tasks that involve coordinating praying together, loved one, primary caregiver, family members. (out of state can be included by speaker phone), on a regular bases.

3. Tasks that coordinate ministries to come to the home and support the primary caregiver as well as the loved one.

4. Support the primary caregiver so they can go on a spiritual retreat.

5. Matters of receiving the sacraments of the Church

6. OTHER: _____

Second Step, Assign Family Members Responsibilities for each Role

Each role has its own responsibility. From this role assignment, a family member takes on a set of responsibilities, then creates their "Plan of Action".

A written "Plan of Action" creates transparency, it identifies where others can provide their assistance in helping to meet the family needs. Each family member should share their plan with the other family members during the quarterly family meeting. A sort of "Report the Progress" will strengthen communications within the family.

A written "Plan of Action" creates clarity of thought. So the right things get done on time with the proper level of focus.

A written "Plan of Action" creates Accountability. Plan your work, work your plan.

 # 1 Financial Role Responsibilities: Assigned To: _____

Gather and organize financial documents in one place. Then, carefully review all documents, even if you're already familiar with them.

1. Paying bills
2. Arranging for benefit claims
3. Making investment decisions
4. Preparing tax returns
5. Financial documents include: Bank and brokerage account information, deeds, mortgage papers or ownership statements
6. Insurance policies
7. Monthly or outstanding bills
8. Pension and other retirement benefit summaries (including VA benefits, if applicable)
9. Rental income paperwork
10. Social Security payment information

Website for more details in managing someone else's money:

http://www.consumerfinance.gov/blog/managing-someone-elses-money/

Paying For Care: (managing bills)

A number of financial resources may be available to help cover the costs of care for the person Alzheimer's Disease or other dementia. Some may apply now and others in the future.

1st Assignment: Become familiar with this web page.

https://www.alz.org/care/alzheimers-dementia-costs-paying-for-care.asp

2nd Assignment https://www.alz.org/care/alzheimers-dementia-financial-legal-planning.asp

CREATING A (Financial Responsibilities) "PLAN OF ACTION" WHO, WIll DO WHAT, HOW IT WILL BE DONE, WHAT REASOURCES ARE NEEDED.
WHEN IT WILL BE COMPLETED

Personal Attache
Organizing Financial, Legal and Medical Records

 # 2 Legal Role Responsibilities: **Assigned To:** _____

Gather and organize Legal documents in one place. Then, carefully review all documents, even if you're already familiar with them.

1. Trust documents
2. Power of Attorney, Healthcare Power of Attorney
3. Will's
4. End of life instructions
5. Burial Plot Purchase
6. Insurance Policies
7. Do Not Resuscitate orders
8. Real Estate documents include: Property Deeds Transfer Up Death, Mortgagees or Promissory Notes, Joint Ownership in Land or Property
9. Personal Property
10. Appraisals
11. Bank Safety Deposit Boxes
12. Memberships and Subscriptions
13. Automatic Payment Bank Withdrawals
14. Website for more details in managing some ones else's legal affairs:
15. Legal Issues in Care: (managing legal affairs)

A number of legal resources may be available to help cover the legal aspects of care for the person Alzheimer's Disease or other dementia. Some may apply now and others in the future.

1st Assignment: https://www.alz.org/national/documents/brochure_legalplans.pdf

CREATING A (Legal Role Responsibilities) "PLAN OF ACTION" WHO, WIll DO WHAT, HOW IT WILL BE DONE, WHAT REASOURCES ARE NEEDED.

Again, keep in mind the primary goal of the roles and responsibilities is to take these assignments off the role of the Primary Caregiver, also to use the gifts and talents that are available from within the family.

Personal Attache
Organizing Financial, Legal and Medical Records

 # 3 Medical Records Role Responsibilities: **Assigned To:** _____

Gather and organize medical documents in one place. Then, carefully review all documents, even if you're already familiar with them.

1. Vital Information
2. Visits to the Doctor
3. Medication Log
4. Medical Consultation Log
5. Doctor Visit
6. Medical Contacts
7. Blood Sugar Tracker
8. Symptoms Tracker
9. Blood Pressure Log
10. Family History
11. Medical Release
12. Dental Log
13. Body Measurements Chart
14. Personal Measurements Charts
15. Vitamin Intake
16. Sleeping Log
17. Journal
18. Lab Results
19. Emergency Room Visits
20. Prescriptions
21. Known Allergies
22. Plan of Treatment
23. Medical Doctor and Staff phone numbers and emails.

Other Services documents include:

☐ Home Healthcare Agency work, PT, OT, Respiratory, Nursing, Medical Supplies, Medical Equipment.

☐ Assisted Living, Rehabilitation Center, Memory Care Unit.

☐ Hospital Stay documents

☐ Home Heath Aid Services

Website for more details in managing some ones else's medical records:

1st Assignment

http://betterhealthwhileaging.net/tools-for-caregivers-keeping-organizing-medical-information/

Paying For Care: (managing bills)
A number of financial resources may be available to help cover the costs of care for the person Alzheimer's Disease or other dementia. Some may apply now and others in the future.

2nd Assignment:
Become familiar with this web page.
https://www.sarahtitus.com/medical-binder/

CREATING A (Medical Records Role Responsibilities) "PLAN OF ACTION" WHO, WIll DO WHAT, HOW IT WILL BE DONE, WHAT REASOURCES ARE NEEDED.

 # 4 Support Network Coordinator Role Responsibilities **Assigned To:** _____

Coordinate and Support the "Support Network". Then, carefully review preparation for upcoming events, and follow up with past events.

1. As a family, set up a support network

2. As a family, set up a support network strategy for each month

3. Determine the resources required to ensure the support network works

4. Handle each participant in the network separately, measure if they are the right entity.

Other Responsibilities include:

- Confirm that Banks, investments, insurance, physicians, home health services, attorneys are all working in the best interest of your loved one.

- Challenge your church to stop by

- Set up and schedule friends to stop by

Personal Attache
Organizing Financial, Legal and Medical Records

- Create a newsletter for updating the network, just the facts.

- Schedule respite outings, overnight breaks

- Laundry and house cleaning support

Website for more details in managing a support network:
http://www.aplaceformom.com/blog/7-19-16-ways-caregivers-can-build-a-support-system/

CREATING A (Support Network Coordinator Role Responsibilities) "PLAN OF ACTION" WHO, WIll DO WHAT, HOW IT WILL BE DONE, WHAT REASOURCES ARE NEEDED.

 # 5 Spirituality Support Coordinator Role Responsibilities Assigned To: _____

Gather and organize resources in practicing your faith. Then, carefully review all documents, even if you're already familiar with them to determine how to best coordinate them into your journey. Be creative.

1. Set up Homebound Eucharistic ministry.
2. Request prayer ministry to make home visit from parish.
3. Parish retreats for your primary Caregiver and family members to attend together.
4. Driving to Mass, someone to watch loved one.

Other Responsibilities include:

- Once each month family gathers to pray rosary together.
- Once a month Skype Divine Mercy chaplet, with family and invited support network.
- First Saturday of the month morning Mass, blessed mother.
- Monthly Adoration, for the primary caregiver to attend, (someone needs to stay and watch your loved one).
- Family Self-Directed Spiritual Development Program.
- http://www.padrepiocleveland.org/   First Saturday each month communion with the Cleveland Padre Pio prayer group, starts with mass, learning and prayer.
- Educate the family on how to use www.formed.org passcode purchased on line at website.

- Educate the family on how to use http://www.usccb.org/bible/readings/Join a local "Legion of Mary" as an Auxiliary member. Look to a parish that has one.
- Purchase from Amazon.com Dementia "Living in the memories of God" John Swinton. View video www.youtube: https://www.youtube.com/watch?v=AvVqhX7E0nU

CREATING A (Spirituality Support Coordinator Role Responsibilities) "PLAN OF ACTION" WHO, WIll DO WHAT, HOW IT WILL BE DONE, WHAT REASOURCES ARE NEEDED.

CHAPTER FOUR:

Designing the Financial Binder

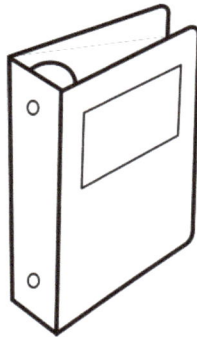

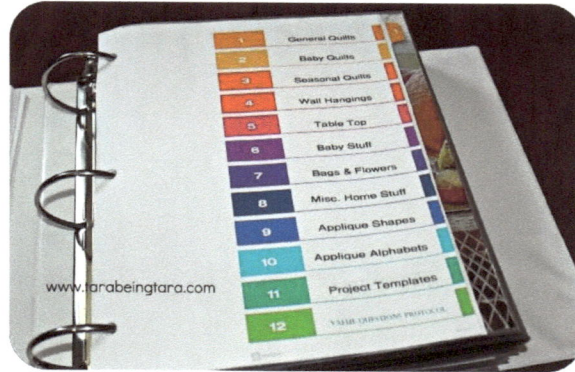

Current Situation Organizing your Financial Estate

Q: Where are your files kept?

Q: Are all the files in one place?

Q: Do you have a functioning file cabinet?

Q: Do you have your contact names and phone numbers in one place, is it up to date and a complete list?

Q: Have you considered using a budget? If Yes, is it working?

Q: Do you have an accountant? When was the last time you spoke?

Q: Do you have a dedicated financial advisor? When was the last time you spoke?

Q: Do you have an attorney? When was the last time you spoke?

Q: What type of housing are you living in? Is it financial sustainable?

Q: In your estate do you have a trust? Is the trust fully funded?

Q: Do you have a will? Are financial assets included?

Q: Do you have real estate investment properties?

Q: Do you own a business or LLC?

Q: Do you have a life insurance policy?

These are the type questions you need to be asking yourself.

Master Financial Assets Inventory

BANK ACCOUNTS: Account Name:	Website	User Name	Passcode	*Account Number:

CREDIT CARD ACCOUNTS: Account Name:	Website	User Name	Passcode	Automatic Withdrawal From Bank Account Name Account Number:

MONTHLY BILLs ACCOUNTS: Account Name: Account Phone Number	Website	User Name	passcode	Automatic Withdrawal From: Account Name Account Number:

On Line Subscriptions: Account Name:	Website	User Name & Passcode	On-line Statement	Automatic Withdrawal From Bank Account Name Account Number:

Personal Attache
Organizing Finance, Legal and Medical Records

Subscriptions/Memberships: Account Name:	Website	User Name & Passcode	On-line Statement	Automatic Withdrawal From Bank Account Name Account Number:

INVESTMENT ACCOUNTS Account Name	Account Address	Point of Contact & Phone Number	Type of Account	*Account Number

Personal Attache
Organizing Financial, Legal and Medical Records

By Asset: Problem Identification Checklist

1# Problem:		Corrective Action Required:	Required Documents:	Comments:
Contact Log Contacted	Date Last	Date Last Contacted:		

#2 Problem:		Corrective Action Required:	Required Documents:	Account Number:
Contact Log Contacted	Date Last	Date Last Contacted:		

#3 Problem:		Corrective Action Required:	Required Documents:	Comments:	Corrective Action Required:
Contact Log Last Contacted	Date	Date Last Contacted:			
Contact Log Last Contacted	Date	Date Last Contacted:			

#4 Problem:		Corrective Action Required:	Required Documents:	Comments:	Corrective Action Required:
Contact Log Last Contacted	Date	Date Last Contacted:			
Contact Log Last Contacted	Date	Date Last Contacted:			
Contact Log Last Contacted	Date	Date Last Contacted:			

Personal Attache
Organizing Financial, Legal and Medical Records

#5 Problem:		Corrective Action Required:	Required Documents:	Comments:	Corrective Action Required:
Contact Log Last Contacted	Date	Date Last Contacted:			
Contact Log Last Contacted	Date	Date Last Contacted:			
Contact Log Last Contacted	Date	Date Last Contacted:			

NOTES ON ACTIVITIES:

_____

_____

_____

_____

_____

_____

_____

_____

_____

_____

_____

_____

_____

CHAPTER FIVE:

Designing the Legal Binder

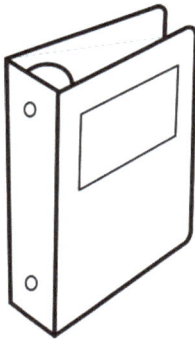
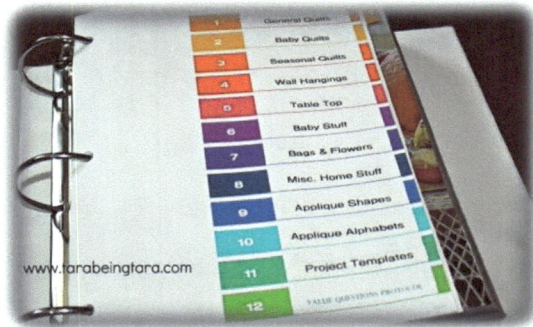

LEARN WHY BEING ORGANIZED IN LEGAL MATTERS, MATTERS.....:

- What is estate planning

- Why is estate planning necessary?

- What happens if I don't have a plan?

- I'm not rich. Do I need an estate plan?

- What's the difference between having a "Will" and a "Living Trust"?

- How does a living trust avoid probate?

- What are the cost benefits of avoiding probate?

- What are the benefits of avoiding probate?

- How will I know whether I need a "Will" or a "Living Trust"?

- What should I consider before I begin estate planning?

- What do I need to accomplish my estate planning goals?

- I already have an estate plan. When should I have it reviewed?

These are the questions that should be answered prior to taking on or assigning roles and responsibilities.

What is estate planning?

Estate planning is the process of working with an attorney who is familiar with your goals, concerns, and assets in order to organize your estate. Estate planning covers the transfer of property at death as well as a variety of personal matters including:

- Choosing beneficiaries

- Care of minor children

- Health care directions

- Power of attorney

- Organ donations

- Burial arrangements

The principal document that is most often associated with this process is your Will.

Why is estate planning necessary?

An effective estate plan ensures that your plans for your medical care, guardianship for minor children, management and distribution of your assets will be carried out according to your wishes and not left to the State of California or others to decide. Estate planning is much more than just having a Will.

What happens if I don't have a plan?

When you die without a Will (a.k.a. "Intestate"), your assets will be distributed according to California State law. Additionally, the Court will appoint guardians for your minor children. Unfortunately, a Probate judge does not know you, your family, or your financial situation better than you. Thus, a judge's decisions about how to divide your assets or who should raise your children may not match your wishes.

Without a valid plan all decisions about your estate must be approved through the Probate Court system, which is very slow and costly process.

I'm not rich....Do I need an plan?

Whether you are rich or poor, young or old, married or single, a parent or without children, you should invest in an estate plan. If you have any of the following:

- Children

- Cash, Stocks, Bonds

- Furniture, Cars, Jewelry

- House

- Business

- Life Insurance

- Social Security Benefits

- Disability

Then you should have an estate plan!

What's the difference between having a "Will" and a "Living Trust"?

A Will is a legal document that specifies how you would like your assets distributed at your death, and who you wish to be the guardians for your minor children. The Will names an executor to facilitate the management of your Will during the Probate process.

A Living Trust, on the other hand, is an estate planning instrument that allows you to maintain greater control over the disposition of your estate and to determine what will happen following your passing. As long as you are alive, you can maintain control over the property in the trust, including using it, selling it, gifting it or spending it.

Upon your passing, the Trust Property may be transferred directly to your heirs, the beneficiaries of the trust, and it will not have to pass through Probate. While you are alive, you will serve as the trustee, and after your passing the trust will fall under the administration of the successor trustee whom you have designated to be the person who manages and distributes the trust property.

Category

Level 1: No Planning

Level 2: Wills

Level 3: Trusts

How it works?

Level 1, State Law dictates who inherits your "estate" (all of your assets) after your

death. Level 2, You specify what happens to your "estate" (all of your assets) after your

death Level 3, You specify what happens to any assets you place in the trust ("trust

property")

Probate?   Level 1, Goes through probate, Level2 Goes through probate Level 3 Avoids probate

Privacy?   Level 1 Public hearing, Level 2 Public hearing, Level 3 Stays private

Beneficiaries? Level 1 Cannot choose who inherits property, Level 2 Names people to inherit your "estate", Level 3 Names people to inherit your "trust property"

Guardians? Level 1 Cannot choose a guardian for your children, Level 2 Names a guardian for your children, Level 3 N/A

Administration? Level 1 Cannot choose an "executor" for your estate, Level 2 Names an "executor" to administer your estate, Level 3 Name yourself as "Trustee" to manage the trust while you are living -Name a "Successor Trustee" to manage the trust after your death

Property Distribution? Level 1 No Control:

-Cannot make specific gifts of property

-Cannot leave assets to step-children, close friends, or charities

-Cannot delay inheritance until beneficiary reaches a certain age

-Cannot control how beneficiaries will use their inheritance

Level 2 Some Control:

-Make specific gifts of property

-State who receives to the rest of your estate (not specifically gifted)

-Entire gift or inheritance goes to beneficiaries (no periodic distributions)

-Cannot delay inheritance until beneficiary reaches a certain age

-Cannot control how beneficiaries will use their inheritance   Max

Level 3 Control and Flexibility:

-Make specific gifts of "trust property"

-State who receives the rest of your trust property (not specifically gifted)

-Make periodic distributions of income or principal

-Make distributions after beneficiaries reach a certain age (21, 25, 30 years old)

-Control how beneficiaries will use their inheritance

Incapacitation? Level 1 May need an expensive conservatorship proceeding, Level 2 May need an expensive conservatorship proceeding, Level 3 Avoids conservatorship à Successor Trustee can manage the trust property if you become incapacitated

Drafting Cost? Level 1None Level 2 $100 - $300 Level 3 $1,000 - $1,500

Probate Cost? Level 1 Extremely High (Avg. $30,000 - $40,000), Level 2

Minimal Level 3 None

How does a Living Trust avoid Probate?

When an estate is conveyed through a Will, the Probate Court must validate the Will before its provisions can be carried out. It can take 12 to 18 months, and typically costs as much as 8-10% of the total value of your estate. Assets held in a Living Trust are not subject to Probate. These assets will pass according to the terms of the Living Trust immediately, without dealing with the cost and delay caused by the Court process.

What are the cost benefits of avoiding Probate?

Probate can be extremely expensive because of Court fees, attorney's fees, executor fees, and appraiser fees. Probate typically costs 8% to 10% of the gross value of the estate.

For example, if your only asset is a $400,000 house, the cost of Probate would be $32,000 to $40,000. But wait....what if there is still $300,000 to pay on the mortgage, reducing your equity to $100,000? The Probate would still cost $32,000 to $40,000, because fees are based on the gross value of your assets, not the actual value.

What are the benefits of avoiding Probate?

Your assets will pass to your beneficiaries faster, more cheaply and privately. For example, your spouse and children could receive income to provide for their living expenses immediately, instead of waiting a 12 to 18 months for Probate Court proceedings to conclude.

How will I know whether I need a "Will" or a "Living Trust"?

After you complete the online interview and/or client intake questionnaire, your information will be reviewed by our attorneys. We will discuss the information with you and decide which course of action best fits your individual circumstances.

What should I consider before I begin estate planning?

- Who will be the executor of your Last Will

- Who will be the successor trustee after you if you draft a Living Trust

- Who should be the Guardian for your minor children

- Who will make financial decisions for you if you cannot make them yourself

- Who will make health care decisions for you if you cannot make them yourself

- How you want your end of life medical care handled

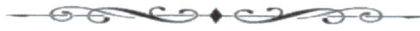

- If you want to make any anatomical gifts at your death

- How you want your estate to be distributed at your death

What do I need to accomplish my estate planning goals?

Estate planning is much more than having a Will. Common estate planning tools include:

- Wills

- Living Trusts

- Powers of Attorney (Financial Decisions)

- Powers of Attorney (Medical Decisions)

- Letters of Instruction

- Beneficiary Designations

When should I have it reviewed?

You should have your estate plan reviewed every 2-3 years. In addition, the following events should trigger an immediate review of your plan:

- the birth of a child

- change in your state of residence

- a significant change in the value or character of your assets

- a change in intended beneficiaries

- the death of a beneficiary

- the death of a guardian, trustee, or personal representative named in your

a change in tax laws affecting federal estate tax deductions and calculations

TRUST

You will need to obtain two notary copies of your trust. In this section you will file a copy of your trust with Notary seal. The original should be kept in a safe deposit box.

Master Legal Asset Inventory

1st Attorney:	Phone:	Stock Broker:	Phone:
	Email:		Email:
	Website:		Website:
2nd Attorney:	Phone:	Accountant CPA:	Phone:
	Email:		Email:
	Website:		Website:

Product Name:	Date Last Updated:	Point of Contact &	Location of	*Account Number:
Healthcare Power of Attorney				
General Power of Attorney				
Living Will				
Advance Directives				
HIPPA Release Form				
Will				
Trust				
Promissory Notes				
Partnerships				

CREATE A LIST THAT BEST MATCHES YOUR PROFILE:

2 Trust(s)
3 Will (s)
4 Probate Plan of Action
5 Financial Power of Attorney
6 Estate Plan of Eldercare
7 Plan for Taxation
8 Master Contact List
9 Birth Certificates
10 Baptismal Certificate
11 Confirmation Certificate
12 Religious Certificates
13 Marriage Certificate (s)
14 Divorce Certificate (s)
15 Annulment Certificate
16 Vehicle Loans

18 Mortgage(s)
19 Auto Insurance Policy
20 Life Insurance Policy
21 Health Insurance Policy
22 Appraisals
23 Promissory Notes
24 Awards
25 Passport(s)
26 Property Deeds
27 Mineral Rights
28 Umbrella Policy
29 Social Security Benefits
30 Employer Retirement Plan
31 Business Ownership Documents

NOTES ON ACTIVITIES:

_____
_____
_____
_____
_____
_____
_____
_____
_____
_____
_____
_____
_____

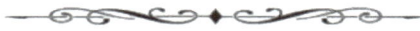

CHAPTER SIX:

Designing the Medical Records Binder

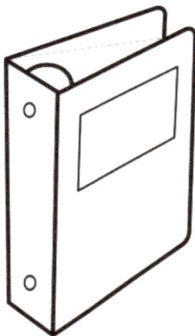

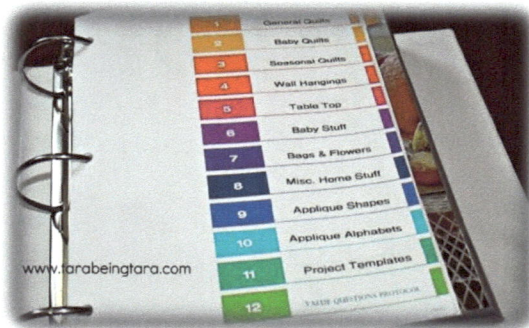

Current Situation Organizing Home Medical Records

Q: Do you have a medical record of your loved ones medications, labs and insurance

documents? Q: Do you have unpaid medical bills?

If yes, How many? How much is the approximate total?

How far back do they go?

Q: What is your loved ones current health status?

Q: To what level does your loved one you receive

aids for daily living?

Q: When was their last hospital admit?

Q: Are you having difficulty working with your insurance company, bill collectors, at home healthcare services?

Q: Do you have any physical limitations?

Medical Organizer Binder and Manual File System

A. The loved ones Medical Records Binder:

    a. To Provide a physician's office or hospital admissions with the necessary information for completing the administrative requirement to provide you medical care services.

    b. To provide a clinical team the general information of your healthcare status.

    c. To facilitate communication in coordination of you healthcare to each critical member of your healthcare team and relatives.

    d. This form should be used during each physician and hospital visit to include the Emergency Room.

B. Medical Business Card Section

    a. Used to retain business cards of the professionals that are providing you care.

C. Physician Office Visit

    a. Used to record current information about your healthcare status

    b. Ask office nursing staff to write in the results for each visit

D. Diagnostic Test Log

    a. For every test there is a numeric result that indicates your status

    b. Keep an updated record of those exact results

    c. Tell you hospital team upon admissions of this chapter in your binder

    d. Let the physician office staff write in your results during your office visit

E. Medications Log

    a. Use this log to record the medications that you are currently taking and have taken in the past.

    b. Under results: state what the drug did for you, this is where you would record the side effects that you experienced while taking this drug

F. Medical Bills and Negotiation

    a. Staying organized with bills is a process.

    b. Have a folder labeled for each account

    c. When the bills come in, place their statements into their accounts

    d. Then plan on returning to these bills

        i. Call the account and get the name of the person in the billing department that negotiates discounts.

        ii. Know the total, the amount that the insurance paid and state 20% as what you are able to pay.

        iii. Try to negotiate all the bills in a single account at the same time.

G. Alternate Site Healthcare Coordination

    a. Use this section to record the critical administration and clinical staff at the facility

    b. Gather these names at the introduction. Go deeper into their organization chart than just the single facility. If a corporation, who are they, where are they headquarters, who at corporate is in charge of clinical operations and C-Level Executives and Legal Councilor.

H. Communication & Coordination Memo (template p.71)

    a. Use Memo template to communicate your concerns to the management and clinical team at the healthcare facility. Copy the same correspondence to the necessary people in their organization.

    b. You can send them this form as your communication or use the form to assemble the facts for what you will include to a letter.

    c. In healthcare, you have to document what is said or it is as if nothing was ever stated. Document, Document, Document.

    d. Do not be afraid to go above someone's head, even the CEO answers to a Board of Trustees, and all of them answer to a government oversight group, State and Federal. But you have to be able to show that you tried to communicate and what the results were for that effort.

Name: Number:		Social Security	Birth Date:	Today's Date:
Address:	Mailing Address: (Same)	Home Phone: Cell Phone:		

My Doctors

Name:	Specialty:	Phone Number:	
1.			
2.			
Height:	Weight: As Of Date:	Color eyes: Color Hair:	

Known Allergies:	Alert Condition:	Blood Type:
1.	2.	3.

List of Medications

Name: Brand/Generic	Dose & Frequency	Date Started

Pre-Existing Conditions, Surgeries or Procedures

Diagnosis	Date/Doctor	Surgeries or Procedures	Date/Doctor

Immunizations Records

Personal Attache

Organizing Financial, Legal and Medical Records

Diagnostic Test Log			
Diagnostic Test Name	Physician Who Ordered Test	Date Of Test	Location of Record for Results

Physician's Name & Specialty Office Visit		
What are my symptoms:	What are my questions	Date of Appt.
		Temperature:
Physician's Diagnosis:		
		BP: /
		Pulse:
		Height:
		Weight:

Physician's Name & Specialty Office Visit		
What are my symptoms:	What are my questions	Date of Appt.
		Temperature:
Physician's Diagnosis:		
		BP: /
		Pulse:
		Height:
		Weight:

Physician's Name & Specialty Office Visit		
What are my symptoms:	What are my questions	Date of Appt.
		Temperature:
Physician's Diagnosis:		
		BP: /
		Pulse:
		Height:
		Weight:

Physician's Name & Specialty		
What are my symptoms:	What are my questions	Date of Appt.
		Temperature:
Physician's Diagnosis:		
		BP: /
		Pulse:
		Height:
		Weight:

Medications Log

Drug Name:	Dose & Frequency:	Date Started:
	Doctor:	Date Stopped:
	Diagnosis:	Result:
	Symptoms to watch out for:	
Drug Name:	Dose & Frequency:	Date Started:
	Doctor:	Date Stopped:
	Diagnosis:	Result:
	Symptoms to watch out for:	
Drug Name:	Dose & Frequency:	Date Started:
	Doctor:	Date Stopped:
	Diagnosis:	Result:
	Symptoms to watch out for:	
Drug Name:	Dose & Frequency:	Date Started:
	Doctor:	Date Stopped:
	Diagnosis:	Result:
	Symptoms to watch out for:	
Drug Name:	Dose & Frequency:	Date Started:
	Doctor:	Date Stopped:
	Diagnosis:	Result:
	Symptoms to watch out for:	
Drug Name:	Dose & Frequency:	Date Started:
	Doctor:	Date Stopped:
	Diagnosis:	Result:
	Symptoms to watch out for:	
Drug Name:	Dose & Frequency:	Date Started:
	Doctor:	Date Stopped:
	Diagnosis:	Result:
	Symptoms to watch out for:	
Drug Name:	Dose & Frequency:	Date Started:
	Doctor:	Date Stopped:
	Diagnosis:	Result:
	Symptoms to watch out for:	
Drug Name:	Dose & Frequency:	Date Started:
	Doctor:	Date Stopped:
	Diagnosis:	Result:

	Dose & Frequency:	
Drug Name:	**Doctor:**	**Date Started:**
	Diagnosis:	**Date Stopped:**
	Symptoms to watch out for:	**Result:**
	Dose & Frequency:	
Drug Name:	**Doctor:**	**Date Started:**
	Diagnosis:	**Date Stopped:**
	Symptoms to watch out for:	**Result:**
	Dose & Frequency:	
Drug Name:	**Doctor:**	**Date Started:**
	Diagnosis:	**Date Stopped:**
	Symptoms to watch out for:	**Result:**
	Dose & Frequency:	
Drug Name:	**Doctor:**	**Date Started:**
	Diagnosis:	**Date Stopped:**
	Symptoms to watch out for:	**Result:**
	Dose & Frequency:	
Drug Name:	**Doctor:**	**Date Started:**
	Diagnosis:	**Date Stopped:**
	Symptoms to watch out for:	**Result:**
	Dose & Frequency:	
Drug Name:	**Doctor:**	**Date Started:**
	Diagnosis:	**Date Stopped:**
	Symptoms to watch out for:	**Result:**
	Dose & Frequency:	
Drug Name:	**Doctor:**	**Date Started:**
	Diagnosis:	**Date Stopped:**
	Symptoms to watch out for:	**Result:**
	Dose & Frequency:	
Drug Name:	**Doctor:**	**Date Started:**
	Diagnosis:	**Date Stopped:**
	Symptoms to watch out for:	**Result:**

Alternate Site Healthcare Coordination

Home Healthcare Agency

Title:	Name:	Phone:	Email:
Director of Nursing			
Respiratory Therapist			
Physical Therapist			
Occupation Therapist			
Speech Therapist			
Manager of Home Health Aids			
Branch Manager			
Regional Director			
Corporate VP Operations			
Physician Certifying This Branch			
Referral Source: Person that referred this organization			

Rehabilitation Center (Out Patient)

Physical Therapy

Title:	Name:	Phone Number:	Email:
Director Of Nursing			
Facility Director			
Physician for Facility			
Supervisor Physical Therapist			
Billing Manager			

Occupation Therapy

Title:	Name:	Phone Number:	Email:
Director Of Nursing			
Facility Director			
Physician for Facility			
Supervisor Physical Therapist			
Billing Manager			

Speech Therapy

Title:	Name:	Phone Number:	Email:
Director Of Nursing			
Facility Director			
Physician for Facility			
Supervisor Physical Therapist			
Billing Manager			

Skilled Nursing Facility (In-Patient)

Title:	Name:	Phone:	Email:	
Director of Nursing				
Shift Supervisor				
Manager Physical Therapy				
Occupation Therapy				
Speech Therapy				

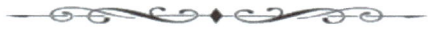

Communication & Coordination Memo

Patient Advocate Name:_____**Relation:** _____
Patient Name:_____**Date:** _____
_____I have,_____Do not have a Healthcare Durable Power of Attorney. Date on File:

Visit Date:	Time of Day:	Talked with Staff, Name:	Reviewed Chart:	Areas of Concern:	Unresolved previous issues:
					See Notes dated:
					See Notes dated:
					See Notes dated:
Corrective Action Has Been Noticed					
1.					
2.					
3.					
4.					
5.					

This Correspondence has been copied to the following: (check if included)

Facility Director: _____   Director of Operations: _____
Facility Medical Director: _____   Patients Physician: _____
Facility Corporate Director or Operations: _____   Facility Corporate General Council: _____
Health Plan Insurance Medical Director: _____   Health Plan, Director of Case Management: _____

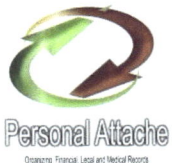

Personal Attache
Organizing Financial, Legal and Medical Records

NOTES ON ACTIVITIES:

_____

_____

_____

_____

_____

_____

_____

_____

_____

_____

_____

_____

_____

CHAPTER SEVEN:

Designing the Support Network Binder

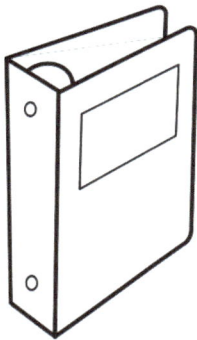

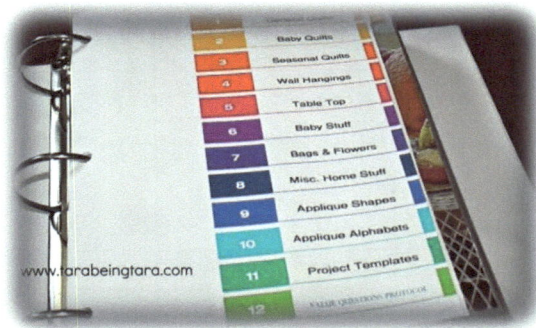

This is a list of "Support Services" that will be used during the Alzheimer's journey. Add to the list as needed

CATEGORY	Primary Point of Contact	Phone:	Email:	Notes:
Active Primary Care Physician				
Neurologist team				
Family Psychiatrist				
Handyman Service				
Social Worker / Case Manager				
Boy Scouts for free yard work				
Private Home Health Aid Company				
City Senior Community Center				
Mail order disposable medical supply company				
Mail order Pharmacy				
Involved Spouse				
Regular Friends				
Local Alzheimer's Association Chapter				

NOTES ON ACTIVITIES:

_____

_____

_____

_____

_____

_____

_____

_____

_____

_____

_____

_____

_____

CHAPTER EIGHT:

Designing the Spiritual Support Binder

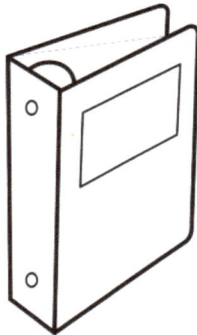

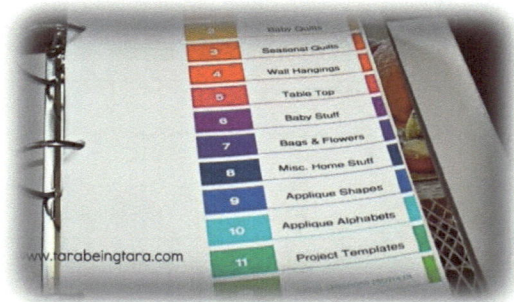

This is a list of spiritual support contacts, according to your faith practices. Add to list as needed.

CATEGORY	Primary Point of Contact:	Phone Number:	Email:	NOTES
Pastor				
Deacon				
Assistant Pastor				
Director Spiritual Ministry				
Senior's Program Leader				
Prayer Group Leader				
Home Eucharistic Ministry				
Pharmacist on team				
Mail order disposable medical supply company				
Mail order Pharmacy				
Involved Spouse				
Regular Friends				
Any disabled dependents in the home				

NOTES ON ACTIVITIES:

_____

_____

_____

_____

_____

_____

_____

_____

_____

_____

_____

_____

CHAPTER NINE:

Designing the Family Plan of Action

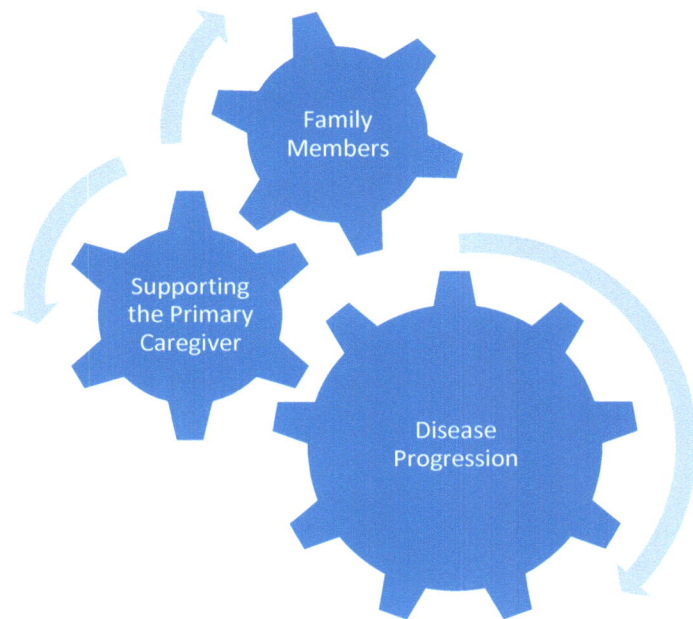

Family Members

Supporting the Primary Caregiver

Disease Progression

Personal Attache
Organizing Financial, Legal and Medical Records

Developing a Family Strategy

Caregiver Strategy: Assess what's has changed?

Status:

What is their current stage in the disease progression?

How long have they been in this stage?

Date for next assessment?
Consider "Now" to be current stage, Future to be "Next Stage"

This strategy will include the behavior and known issues which are likely to present in the next stage.

1. **Changes to Expect with Your Family Member or Friend**

Now:

_____

_____

Future:

_____

_____

2. **Caregiving Strategies for Any Activity**

Now:

_____

_____

Future:

_____

_____

3. **Your Role as a Primary Caregiver and How you will Cope in the next stage**

Now:

_____

_____

Future:

_____

_____

4. **Orientation, What Changes to Expect**

Now:

_____

_____

Future:

_____

_____

5. **The loved one's communication and language changes to expect**

Now:

_____

_____

Future:

_____

_____

6. Emotional and Behavioral Changes To Expect

Now:

_____

_____

Future:

_____

_____

7. Independence and Basic Care

Now:

_____

_____

Future:

_____

_____

8. Travel and Movement

Now:

_____

_____

Future:

_____

_____

9. Finances and Shopping

Now:

_____

_____

Future:

_____

_____

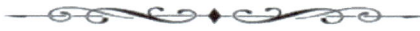

10. Preparing Food and Eating

Now:

_____

_____

Future:

_____

_____

11. Managing Medication

Now:

_____

_____

Future:

_____

_____

12. Using the Telephone

Now:

_____

_____

Future:

_____

_____

13. Work and Leisure

Now:

_____

_____

Future:

_____

_____

14. Summary of Information About This Level

Now:

_____

_____

Future:

_____

_____

NOTES ON ACTIVITIES:

_____

_____

_____

_____

_____

_____

_____

_____

_____

_____

_____

_____

CHAPTER TEN:

Appendix(s)

APPENDIX ONE:

The Alzheimer's Family Initial Meeting Agenda

Agenda

"Family Meeting"

Location:

Time:

1. Identify the stage and what was discovered in the most resent assessment

2. Gain a consensus of the work that is needed for the next 4 months

3. Review Family roles and current projects/tasks

4. Use the Decision-Making Model for the family, what decisions are needed

5. Review a list of known Critical Issues to consider, current stage and the next stage

6. Discuss action items that may be required in the near future

7. Roles and Responsibilities Assignments, progress report

8. Create a Plan of Action for the next 4 months

9. Determine date for follow up meeting

Identifying Your Family Values

Family Values

In Values, we find ourselves taking a stance on how we will follow a certain way towards making a decision. It is therefore important to understand the family values, prior to making critical decisions about the lives of our loved one.

Values (ethics)

From Wikipedia, the free encyclopedia

In ethics, **values** denotes the degree of importance of some thing or action, with the aim of determining what actions are best to do or what way is best to live (normative ethics), or to describe the significance of different actions (axiology). It may be described as treating actions themselves as abstract objects, putting value to them. It deals with right conduct and good life, in the sense that a highly, or at least relatively highly, valuable action may be regarded as ethically "good" (adjective sense), and an action of low in value, or somewhat relatively low in value, may be regarded as "bad.

What do you treasure the most that is without substitution for anything else? Write them down as individual family members.

1.

2.

3.

Now discuss them together as a family, each person stating what they feel are your family values. (note: there is no wrong answer).

Our Family Values Are:

1.

2.

3.

Personal Attache
Organizing Financial, Legal and Medical Records

Family Decision Making Model

"15. Let the peace of Christ rule in your hearts, since as members of one body you were called to peace. And be thankful. 16. Let the message of Christ dwell among you richly as you teach and admonish one another with all wisdom through psalms, hymns, and songs from the Spirit, singing to God with gratitude in your hearts. 17. And whatever you do, whether in word or deed, do it all in the name of the Lord Jesus, giving thanks to God the Father through him." Colossians 3:15-17New International Version (NIV)

PURPOSE: The purpose of a family meeting is multi-faceted. It can serve to communicate information regarding the loved one's situation, or the status of family members. The meeting can also be used to make critical decisions or to determine role responsibilities. In many cases it is all of these.

TASK: In order to make effective decisions as a group, an agreed upon process is important to ensure participation and success in making the best decision. As a family, you are tasked to make many decisions in the Alzheimer's journey. This model will provide a frame work that when used will be helpful to gain the best insight to the problem, create a criteria of importance, consider the options and weigh the possible outcomes.

CONDITION: By gathering as a group to learn about the Alzheimer's disease and its related progression, and dementia behavior, the family has taken the first step in making strong decisions. The second step is to understand the stages and dementia related behavior that will occur. In the final step by gathering as a family, review the family values, understand how to use a "Family Decision Model", assigning Roles and Responsibilities. Then set-up a strategy for the next few months. These are all great steps towards self-empowerment.

STANDARD: The standard is that each person will participate. The individual family member will take on an assigned role and be responsible to achieve that assignment in that role to their best ability. They will seek assistance when needed and give willingly when asked. Each family member will proactively be involved in decisions and communication with respect, dignity and a positive, "Can Do" attitude.

Using Values Based Decision Making Decisions

In Value Based Decision Making, we find ourselves taking a stance on how we will follow a certain way towards making a decision. It is therefore important to understand the family values, prior to making critical decisions about the lives of our loved one.

Values (ethics)

From Wikipedia, the free encyclopedia

In ethics, **values** denotes the degree of importance of some thing or action, with the aim of determining what actions are best to do or what way is best to live (normative ethics), or to describe the significance of different actions (axiology). It may be described as treating actions themselves as abstract objects, putting value to them. It deals with right conduct and good life, in the sense that a highly, or at least relatively highly, valuable action may be regarded as ethically "good" (adjective sense), and an action of low in value, or somewhat relatively low in value, may be regarded as "bad.

Write down your top three values, those you feel are the families.

Each family member reads what they wrote down.

Where there were alike values, make a list.

Determine, which of this list are the top three values for your family.

Write down which the family agrees are your families top three values. Prioritize them 1-3.

Our Family Values Are:
1.
2.
3.

Take the final list of the families top three values and use them in this "decision Making Model"

Personal Attache
Organizing Financial, Legal and Medical Records

DECISION MAKING MODEL

First Step: Identify Exactly What Happened

Exercise: What Happened?

Identify the details of the situation? (what happened, how did it happen, who was involved?)
What:_____
_____
_____
_____How:_____
_____
_____
_____Who:_____
_____
_____
_____

Identify what you would have like to have happened?
_____
_____
_____
_____
_____
_____
_____
_____
_____
_____
_____
_____

Second Step: Analyzing the Situation

Every problem has a situation that surrounds it. Inside the situation is where you will find the solution to the problem. By analyzing the situation more closely, the solution will typically present itself. It will then be clarified and used in your decision-making process.

Exercise: We will take a look at the problem that impacts the situation. (what went wrong)

1 Assessing the Problem: (Describe exactly what is happening that is not working?)

_____

_____

_____

_____

2 Identify, what is causing this to happen?

_____
_____
_____
_____

3 In what areas did this create an impacting or disruption?

_____

_____

_____

_____

_____

_____

Third Step: What is the number one contributing factor?

_____

_____

_____

_____

_____

Fourth Step: Gathering Information

It may seem unnecessary to have a segment that reviews "Gathering Information" however, this is a critical part of the decision-making process and can significantly impact the quality of your decision and its outcome.

There are three types of information to consider gathering:
1. The Primary Source information, The person it happened to, or from someone that was there.
2. The Secondary Source information, He Said She Said.
3. The Gut Feeling Source, no one person saw it happen, but I think this is what occurred.

All of the above information types are reasonable to include in the decision-making model.

The Primary Source: Prepare a list of questions and then go to the primary source for answers. At times you may not know which questions are best to ask. So, research possible questions, then go ask them.

For Example: If you are considering moving your loved one into a facility, go to the facility and take a tour. Do not just read their website, listen to someone else's opinion about the facility or telephone them for a few answers. You will need to go directly to them as they are the "primary source" of information. You should come with a prepared list of questions in order to have an accurate understanding of their facility.

The Secondary Source: This is also a good resource to consider using when making a decision. The Secondary source is valuable because it allows others to provide information about your search for answers. From Secondary Sources you may find other topics or questions that need to be considered.

There are two areas that you need to be aware of; 1. The source of the secondary information. Who are they, what authority do they speak from, why are they providing this information. 2. Is this information a direct correlation to the topic that you are researching. Be careful, sometimes in secondary search it becomes tempting to seek out information that proves your premises to be correct. That is called bias. We want to avoid being bias, just the facts please.

The Gut Feeling: This is a combination of your past experiences, your family upbringing, your spiritualty, and your cultural values and beliefs. They are all wrapped into one feeling of an emotional response. It should not be ignored and rarely should it be the only information feedback that is used in making an informed "Values Based Decision".

Third: Identifying Reasonable Options

The process of identifying reasonable options can only come after you understand the problem, considered your values, reviewed some of the considerations and circumstances as you continue to gather more information.

Once you completed the information gathering phase of *decision making process*, it is at this point when you will eliminate ideas that are not a good fit and consider only those ideas that will work best. Use your values when considering options, use prayer for guidance, let the Holy Spirit take charge and follow what you believe God would have you do. It is our will to do His will.

Exercise: What are the top three pieces of gathered information?

INFORMATION GATHERING CARD

Gathered Information:

_____

_____

_____

_____

Personal Attache
Organizing Financial, Legal and Medical Records

Fifth Step: Criteria for Solution

Exercise: Does your solution qualify for consideration?

CRITICAL CRITERIA, *final Review*

1. Will this action ensure safety for your loved one?   __T_F
2. Do you have the resources needed to complete these tasks?   __T ___F
3. Is your time table realistic?   __T ___F
4. Do you understand the negative impact(s) your actions may create?   __T ___F
5. Would you want others to take this action on your behalf?   __T ___F

Sixth Step: Choose Best Solution

Exercise: Take your decision and place it here:

_____

_____

_____

_____

_____

_____

We will do the following:

_____

_____

_____

_____

_____

_____

Our expected outcome is:

_____

_____

_____

_____

_____

_____

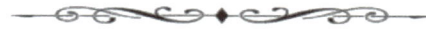

APPENDIX TWO:

Pre-Funeral Set Up

SECTION 1: BASIC INFORMATION

Personal Information

Name (Last)_____(First)_____(Middle)

_____

Suffix (e.g., Sr., Jr.)_____Sex (M / F)_____Social Security No. _____

Citizenship (country)_____Ancestry _____

Ethnic Group/Race_____Religion _____

Residence

Residential

Street Address_____Apt./Unit #_____Facility Name _____

City_____County_____State _____

Zip_____Country _____

Birth Information

Date of Birth_____City of Birth _____

County_____State_____Country _____

Emergency Information

Person to Contact Phone _____

Physician Phone _____

Persons to be Notified

Name_____Address_____Phone _____

Name_____Address_____Phone _____

Name_____Address_____Phone _____

Name_____Address_____Phone _____

Notifications, continued

Contacts for Legal Matters

Person Responsible for Funeral Arrangements

Name_____Phone _____

Address_____City_____State_____Zip _____

Attorney

Name_____Firm_____Phone _____

Address_____City_____State_____Zip _____

Executor of Estate

Firm Name_____Phone _____

Address_____City_____State_____Zip _____

Obituary

Newspaper(s) _____

Other _____

Identify where the following important documents are located:

- ☐ Will
- ☐ Birth Certificate
- ☐ Marriage License
- ☐ Social Security Card
- ☐ Citizenship papers, if appropriate
- ☐ Military Discharge Papers
- ☐ Life and Other Insurance Policies
- ☐ Deeds and Titles to Property (home, autos, etc)
- ☐ Bank Account Passbooks
- ☐ Income Tax Returns
- ☐ Certificates of Ownership of Burial Property
- ☐ Bills to be Paid and other Financial Information
- ☐ Location of Safe Deposit Box
- ☐ Financial Institution Phone
- ☐ Address City State Zip

Choose method of final disposition:

Whole body burial or entombment

Cremation

Specify disposition of ashes:

Burial or entombment at cemetery Scattering at cemetery

Deliver to survivors Other

Donation to medical science

Specify Recipient Organization, if one has been selected:

Organization

Address

City/State/Zip

Telephone

Other: Specify_____(e.g., burial at sea, scatter in outer space)

Also specify the Service Provider, if one has been selected:

Organization

Address

City/State/Zip

Telephone

SECTION 2: DETAILED FUNERAL SERVICE INFORMATION

Choose a type of Funeral Service Plan:
Traditional (includes a visitation and a funeral service in which the deceased is present in an open or closed casket)

Memorial (includes one or more services without the presence of the deceased)

Graveside (includes one service held at the graveside prior to interment)

Traditional Plus (includes a visitation and a funeral service in which the deceased is present in an open or closed casket, plus one or more memorial services without the presence of the deceased)
Direct (the deceased is buried, cremated or donated to medical science without any funeral services)

Select the following services regarding preparation and care:

Do you want to have an embalming performed? (Y/N)_____(this may be required)

Do you want a DNA sample taken? (Y/N) _____

Do you want an autopsy performed? (Y/N)_____(this may be required)

Casket Presentation Selections

- Select how you prefer the casket presented at the visitation(s): Open Closed

- Select how you prefer the casket presented at the funeral: Open Closed

- Do you want only a private family viewing? (Y/N) _____

Note: the deceased will be dressed and cosmetics will be applied if you have chosen to have a private family viewing or select to have an open casket presentation. If you do not wish to have the deceased dressed and cosmeticized for viewings, please explain below how you would like the deceased to be presented:

Clothing Selections

New

Existing

Jewelry

Clothing Selections to be made by:

(Make these selections if a Traditional or Traditional Plus Service Plan has been chosen)

Choose a location for the visitation:

Funeral Home

Church, temple, synagogue or other religious sanctuary Other Facility (describe) _____

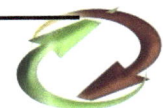

Personal Attache
Organizing Financial, Legal and Medical Records

Visitation Selections, continued

Indicate name, address and telephone of chosen location:

Name

Address

City_____State_____Zip

Telephone_____Fax _____

Choose method of transporting the deceased between service locations and to the cemetery

Funeral Coach or Hearse

Funeral Van (more economical)

Choose method of transporting family members between service locations and to the cemetery

Limousine # of people _____

Sedan # of people _____

Family will provide transportation

Escort Needed? (Y/N)_____Instructions _____

Service Selections

Indicate type of Service:

Funeral Service Memorial Service

Choose a location for the funeral service:

Funeral Home

Church, temple, synagogue or other religious sanctuary

Other Facility (specify) _____

Funeral / Memorial Service Selections, continued

Indicate name, address and telephone of chosen location:

Name Address

City State_____Zip

Telephone Fax

Clergy Presiding

Name_____Affiliation_____Phone _____

Name_____Affiliation_____Phone _____

Name_____Affiliation_____Phone _____

Pallbearers

(Make these selections if a Traditional or Traditional Plus or Graveside Service Plan has been selected)

Active, Honorary

or Alternate?

Name_____Phone _____

Name_____Phone _____

Name_____Phone _____

Name_____Phone _____

Name_____Phone _____

Name_____Phone _____

Name_____Phone _____

Name_____Phone _____

Music

Title_____Artist _____

Title_____Artist _____

Title_____Artist _____

Title_____Artist _____

Title_____Artist _____

Funeral / Memorial Service Selections, continued

Performers

Organist Name_____Phone _____

Vocalist Name_____Phone _____

_____Name_____Phone _____

_____Name_____Phone _____

_____Name_____Phone _____

Readings

Title_____Source/Reference

To be read by:_____Phone

Title_____Source/Reference

To be read by:_____Phone

Title_____Source/Reference

To be read by:_____Phone

Title_____Source/Reference

To be read by:_____Phone

Flowers

Florist Phone

Floral Selection #1

Floral Selection #2

Floral Selection #3

Floral Selection #4

Funeral / Memorial Service Selections, continued

Memorial displays

Description _____

_____

_____

Special Service Components

(Complete this section to provide instructions for special service components such as a 21-gun salute, horse-drawn

procession, or

the rites of fraternal organizations like Masonic organizations or Veterans of Foreign Wars)

Description _____

_____

Floral

Masses

Charitable

Preferred Charity #1:_____Telephone

Address:_____City/State/Zip:

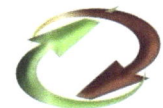

Preferred Charity #2:_____Telephone

Address:_____City/State/Zip:

(Complete this section if a burial or scattering at the cemetery has been chosen)

Cemetery Name Address

City_____State_____Zip _____

Telephone_____Fax _____

Property Identification:

Garden Lot_____Space _____

Niche (for urn)

SECTION 3: DETAILED FUNERAL MERCHANDISE INFORMATION

Casket

Manufacturer_____Model #_____Model Name _____

Identify type of casket:

Wood Specify_____(e.g., birch, cherry, mahogany, maple, oak, pine, poplar, walnut, etc.)

Precious Metal Specify_____(bronze or copper) Sealed? (Y/N) _____

Steel Specify_____(16, 18 or 20 gauge) Stainless? (Y/N)_____Sealed? (Y/N) _____

Cloth covered

Other Specify _____

Identify lid style:

Half Couch (2 piece) Full Couch (1 piece)

Identify interior features:

Material_____(e.g., crepe, linen, velour, velvet) Color _____

Style_____(e.g., shirred, tailored, tufted)

Special Features _____

Outer Burial Container

Manufacturer_____Model #_____Model Name _____

Identify type of outer burial container:

Grave Box or Grave Liner Specify_____(e.g., concrete or wood)

Vault Specify_____(e.g., bronze, copper, concrete, plastic, wood, composite)

Lawn Crypt Specify_____(e.g., concrete or wood)

Special Features _____

Funeral Merchandise, continued

Cremation Urn

Manufacturer_____Model #_____Model Name _____

Material_____(e.g., bronze, ceramic, marble, wood)

Grave Marker

Manufacturer_____Model #_____Model Name _____

Identify type of grave marker:

Grave Marker (flush to the ground) Specify_____(e.g., bronze, granite, marble)

Monument (upright) Specify_____(e.g., bronze, granite, marble)

Lawn Crypt Specify_____(e.g., concrete or wood)

Engraving

_____

Stationery Products

Guest Register Book: Manufacturer_____Style_____Quantity _____

Prayer Cards: Manufacturer_____Style_____Quantity _____

Verse to print on Prayer Cards: _____

Memorial Folders: Manufacturer_____Style_____Quantity _____

Verse to print on Memorial Folders _____

Prayer Books: Manufacturer_____Style_____Quantity _____

Acknowledgement Cards: Manufacturer_____Style_____Quantity _____

_____Manufacturer_____Style_____Quantity _____

SECTION 4: ADDITIONAL PERSONAL INFORMATION

Marital Information

Marital Status (single / married / widowed / divorced) _____

Spouse

Name (Last)_____(First)_____(Middle) _____

Suffix (e.g., Sr., Jr.)_____Sex (M / F)_____Social Security No. _____

Living? (Y/N)_____Birth Date_____Date of Death _____

Address_____City_____State_____Zip _____

Country_____Telephone_____E-Mail _____

Marriage Data

Date of Marriage_____City_____State_____Country _____

Parents

Father Data

Name (Last)_____(First)_____(Middle) _____

Suffix (e.g., Sr., Jr.)_____Living? (Y/N)_____Date of Death _____

Birth Date_____Birth Place _____

Married (Y/N)_____Spouse Name (if not Mother) _____

Address_____City_____State_____Zip _____

Country_____Telephone_____E-Mail _____

Mother Data

Name (Last)_____(First)_____(Middle) _____

Maiden Name_____Living? (Y/N)_____Date of Death _____

Birth Date_____Birth Place _____

Married (Y/N)_____Spouse Name (if not Father) _____

Address_____City_____State_____Zip _____

Country_____Telephone_____E-Mail _____

Additional Personal Information, continued

Children

Child #1

Name (Last)_____(First)_____(Middle) _____

Suffix (e.g., Sr., Jr.)_____Male/Female (M/F) _____

Living? (Y/N)_____Birth Date_____Date of Death _____

Married? (Y/N)_____Spouse Name_____No. of Children _____

Address_____City_____State_____Zip _____

Country_____Telephone _____

E-Mail _____

Child #2

Name (Last)_____(First)_____(Middle) _____

Suffix (e.g., Sr., Jr.)_____Male/Female (M/F) _____

Living? (Y/N)_____Birth Date_____Date of Death _____

Married? (Y/N)_____Spouse Name_____No. of Children _____

Address_____City_____State_____Zip _____

Country_____Telephone _____

E-Mail _____

Child #3

Name (Last)_____(First)_____(Middle) _____

Suffix (e.g., Sr., Jr.)_____Male/Female (M/F) _____

Living? (Y/N)_____Birth Date_____Date of Death _____

Married? (Y/N)_____Spouse Name_____No. of Children _____

Address_____City_____State_____Zip _____

Country_____Telephone _____

E-Mail _____

Additional Personal Information, continued

Siblings

Brother/Sister #1

Name (Last)_____(First)_____(Middle) _____

Suffix (e.g., Sr., Jr.)_____Male/Female (M/F) _____

Living? (Y/N)_____Birth Date_____Date of Death _____

Married? (Y/N)_____Spouse Name_____No. of Children _____

Address_____City_____State_____Zip _____

Country_____Telephone _____

E-Mail _____

Brother/Sister #2

Name (Last)_____(First)_____(Middle) _____

Suffix (e.g., Sr., Jr.)_____Male/Female (M/F) _____

Living? (Y/N)_____Birth Date_____Date of Death _____

Married? (Y/N)_____Spouse Name_____No. of Children _____

Address_____City_____State_____Zip _____

Country_____Telephone _____

E-Mail _____

Brother/Sister #3

Name (Last)_____(First)_____(Middle) _____

Suffix (e.g., Sr., Jr.)_____Male/Female (M/F) _____

Living? (Y/N)_____Birth Date_____Date of Death _____

Married? (Y/N)_____Spouse Name_____No. of Children _____

Address_____City_____State_____Zip _____

Country_____Telephone _____

E-Mail _____

Grandchildren

No. of Grandchildren_____No. of Great Grandchildren_____No. of Great-Great Grandchildren _____

Additional Personal Information, continued

History of Residences

City / State / Country_____No. of Years _____

City / State / Country_____No. of Years _____

City / State / Country_____No. of Years _____

City / State / Country_____No. of Years _____

Education

Elementary School City/State

High School City/State

Year Graduated _____

Undergraduate College City/State

Undergraduate Degree_____Year _____

Graduate College City/State

Graduate Degree_____Year _____

Military Record

Branch of Service_____Years Served From_____To _____

Rank_____Service Number _____

Wars Served_____Decorations _____

Work History

Retired? (Y/N)_____Year Retired _____

Principle occupation_____No. of Years _____

Industries _____

Secondary occupation_____No. of Years _____

Industries _____

Employer #1_____City/State _____

Years From_____To _____

Employer #2_____City/State _____

Years From_____To _____

Additional Personal Information, continued

Employer #3_____City/State _____

Years From_____To _____

Employer #4_____City/State _____

Years From_____To _____

Religious Institutions

Institution #1 _____

Institution #2 _____

Memberships and Public Offices Held

Organization #1_____Position(s) Held _____

Organization #2_____Position(s) Held _____

Organization #3_____Position(s) Held _____

Organization #4_____Position(s) Held _____

Organization #5_____Position(s) Held _____

Notable Accomplishments

Accomplishment #1

_____

_____

Accomplishment #2

_____

_____

Accomplishment #3

_____

_____

Accomplishment #4

_____

APPENDIX THREE:

Pre-Probate Preparation

The family, in preparation of completing probate needs to:

CONTACT INFORMATION

- ☐ lawyer and executor of your will
- ☐ accountant, CPA, and bookkeeper
- ☐ stock broker, investment counselor, and financial advisor
- ☐ insurance agents (life, home, auto, etc.)
- ☐ business associates and partners
- ☐ family, friends, and colleagues

DOCUMENT LOCATOR

- ☐ legal (wills, powers of attorney, trust documents, safe deposit box)
- ☐ family (birth, adoption, guardianship, citizenship, marriage, divorce)
- ☐ banking (loans, list of accounts, statements, cancelled checks, passbooks)
- ☐ investments (CD, securities, stocks, bonds, retirement, annuities)
- ☐ business (incorporation papers, contracts, agreements, computer back-up)
- ☐ deeds and titles (title insurance, property, home inventory, vehicles)
- ☐ insurance (life, death benefits, property, health, homeowners, auto)
- ☐ military (service records, discharge, pension)
- ☐ ID (passport, driver's license, social security card)
- ☐ income tax records

PLANNING IN ADVANCE

- ☐ Have you outlined your funeral arrangements and burial plans?
- ☐ Have you purchased a cemetery plot?
- ☐ Have you purchased a pre-paid funeral or cremation plan?
- ☐ Have you selected the music, prayers, and readings for your service?
- ☐ Have you made it known what you don't want to happen at your service?
- ☐ i.e. religious prayers, open casket viewing, etc.

Personal Attache
Organizing Financial, Legal and Medical Records

TAKING CARE OF YOUR LOVED ONES

- ☐ Have you set up guardianship papers for your children? (if required)
- ☐ Do you know how much money your family needs to replace your income?
- ☐ Do you have adequate current life insurance to cover your family's needs?
- ☐ Do you have enough money specifically set aside to pay the cost of dying?
- ☐ including inheritance taxes, executor, and probate fees
- ☐ Do you have money set aside or LTC insurance for long-term medical costs?
- ☐ Do you have beneficiaries for your accounts, investments, and insurance?

TAXES

- ☐ Have you set up a trust to protect your assets from undue taxation?
- ☐ Do you know how much inheritance tax will be due on your assets?
- ☐ Do you know how much it will cost to have your will probated?
- ☐ Have you left assets to your spouse which can be received tax-free?
- ☐ Have you begun gifting tax-free money to your children prior to your death?
- ☐ Are you planning to make a charitable gift as part of your estate plan?

YOUR WISHES

- ☐ Do you have a current, up-to-date, signed will?
- ☐ Do you have a financial power of attorney set up?
- ☐ Do you have a living will and medical power of attorney?
- ☐ Do you have a current signed organ donor card?
- ☐ Have you given copies of these documents to your executor and attorney?
- ☐ Have you clearly outlined how you want your possessions distributed?
- ☐ Have you labeled any items you want to go to specific people?

Death and Finances: Eight Things to Do After a Loved One Passes Away
by Lynnette Khalfani-Cox Feb 14th 2011

Dealing with the death of a loved one is stressful enough. But not knowing what to do with someone's finances after the person has passed away poses an additional burden on a grieving family.

To make the process a bit easier, here's a checklist of the top eight money matters you must deal with -- and mistakes to avoid -- after someone you care about dies. This checklist isn't all-inclusive. But what follows is critical information that can save you precious time, money and energy, as well as help you avoid squabbles over assets or financial exploitation.

1. Get Multiple Copies of the Death Certificate

If you are the spouse or executor/executrix of the deceased person, the first order of business is to go to the city clerk's office or your local vital statistics office and get certified copies of the death certificate. Obtain at least 10 copies; 20 copies would be even better.

Here's why: A dizzying number of financial institutions, government agencies, creditors, unions, membership groups and other organizations won't even talk to you about a loved one's financial affairs -- let alone take action, like closing an account -- until you produce a death certificate. So you'll need this valuable document before you start contacting banks, investment companies and other firms.

There's another reason to immediately request multiple death certificates. "Nobody is going to pay you anything without them," says insurance agent Al Canton, owner of A.N. Canton Insurance Services, in Fair Oaks, Calif.
The cost of getting a single certified copy of a death certificate typically ranges from about $5 to $20. But additional certified copies are often provided at a discount if you order them with your initial request. Also, many funeral homes will give you one or two certified copies of the death certificate free of charge.

2. Obtain Letters Testamentary or Letters of Administration

Before you can reach out to institutions that a deceased person was doing business with, you'll have to provide those companies with proof that you have a right to wrap up the deceased's financial affairs.

The proof you need is in the form of documents called letters testamentary, or letters of administration.

If you retain an attorney (more info on that below), he or she can secure these documents for you and help you navigate probate court, among other things. For those who decide to go it alone, here's how you get the letters testamentary.

If the person who passed away had a will and you are the executor of the estate, you can obtain letters testamentary from the local courthouse or city hall in the county where the deceased was living when he or she died. You must take the official will to the court, along with a certified death certificate, and file a probate petition.

Once the court opens a probate file and validates the will, it gives you the authority (via the letters testamentary) to carry out the duties required to settle the estate and act on behalf of the deceased, in accordance with the person's will. (As with death certificates, be sure to get multiple certified copies of letters testamentary).

If no will was left behind, the court can issue letters of administration to a surviving spouse or next of kin after a death certificate has been supplied. In this instance, the person to whom letters of administration are issued is deemed the administrator of the estate.

"Whomever is put in charge of the estate or trust should encourage open communication among the beneficiaries," says legacy attorney Andrew Mayoras. Mayoras and his wife, Danielle, are estate planning specialists who co-wrote the book Trial and Heirs: Famous Fortune Fights.

Andrew says that most estate disputes can almost always be traced to a lack of communication. "Secrecy creates doubts," he says, "and sometimes that turns into fights."

3. Consult a Lawyer – Even if You Decide Not to Hire One

After a loved one dies, many heirs balk at hiring legal help because they worry about the cost.

But that's often a penny wise and a pound foolish since advice from a qualified professional could save an estate many thousands of dollars, make the process of settling an estate much easier and help family members avoid potential liabilities.

"When you act as executor, there is fiduciary liability and exposure to you personally if you do not follow the terms of the will exactly," notes estate attorney Rebecca Doane.

For instance, "executors can be surcharged [fined] if they distribute funds improperly," says Doane, who is the founder of Doane & Doane, P.A., an estate planning firm based in North Palm Beach, Fla. A good lawyer will help you sidestep this pitfall.

Aside from wanting to understand possible liability issues, some people may simply be too emotionally overwhelmed do everything alone. "I've had adult children who've graduated from Ivy League business schools who are so grief-stricken that they come in and say 'I can't handle this,' " says Doane, adding that there's no shame in asking for help. Seeking professional support is a good idea, even if only to get a free consultation about your family's situation.

If you do retain an attorney, hire one who handles wills, trusts and estates exclusively. Avoid real estate lawyers, divorce lawyers, personal injury or criminal attorneys, and others who don't specialize in estate planning. And only select a board-certified attorney. Ideally, try to work with a lawyer or firm that is AV rated. That indicates the attorney or firm has received the highest possible professional standards and ethics rankings.

Personal Attache
Organizing Financial, Legal and Medical Records

4. Collect and Secure Pertinent Documents

One of the most time-consuming aspects of tending to the financial affairs of someone who has passed away is gathering the litany of documents that need to be assembled. For many families, this is a nightmare chore due to haphazard record-keeping, poor planning and a lack of knowledge about where critical documents are located.

"A lot of people think that estate planning is only for someone who's old or who has lots of money. But that's not true," says attorney Danielle Mayoras, co-founder of The Center for Probate Litigation.

That's why Mayoras and other experts suggest that while people are alive, they should create an inventory or list of all assets, accounts and property, put that list in a safe place, and then tell a trusted confidante where the list is kept.

After a person's death, an executor of an estate should collect or order the following documents, at a minimum:
- the death certificate(s)
- the will or trust
- insurance policies (life, homeowners, health, disability, auto, etc.)
- last credit card statements
- investment accounts (IRAs, 401(k) plans, mutual funds, pensions, etc.)
- last checking and savings account statements (including CDs and money-market accounts)
- last mortgage statement
- last two years' tax returns
- marriage and birth certificates (of the deceased's spouse and children)
- an up-to-date credit report of the deceased

All these documents will help you find accounts and assets, and assess outstanding debts, as well as submit claims for benefits and cash payments that may be due the deceased person's beneficiaries and heirs.

5. Notify Financial Institutions, Government Agencies and Others

A key next step is to notify all the following places of the individual's death. Each is important for different reasons.
- Social Security Administration
- The deceased person's employer
- Insurance companies
- Credit bureaus
- Credit card companies

- Post office
- Utility companies
- Creditors

It's not much, but Social Security does offer survivors a $255 one-time death benefit. More importantly, the spouse or children of someone who dies may be eligible for monthly survivor benefits from Social Security. To find out if you qualify, contact Social Security online or call 800-772-1213.

Another reason to notify Social Security is so the agency can put the deceased person on the Social Security Master Death Index. This prevents would-be fraudsters from collecting a dead person's Social Security payments. It also helps stop identity thieves from opening accounts in the name of the deceased individual, because the person's credit reports will be flagged.

"Every creditor also needs to know right away because the last thing you want is for bills to continue to run," says Adam Levin, a former director of the New Jersey Division of Consumer Affairs. Prompt notification of the death to various businesses, adds Levin, "saves the estate money and protects the estate of the deceased."

Levin also suggests contacting the Direct Marketing Association to opt the deceased person out of receiving credit solicitations. "You don't want them getting pre-approved credit card offers or convenience checks tied to credit cards," Levin notes.

The U.S. Postal Service doesn't have to be told per se that the individual has died. Rather, you should file a change of address with the postal service, so that mail is rerouted to the executor of the estate or to a trusted family member.

6. Cancel or Transfer Accounts, Memberships and Subscriptions

Following someone's death, you don't want subscriptions, memberships or services they'll no longer be using to stay in force. So cancel those immediately, along with credit card, insurance and financial accounts that will be inactive. "If the person was married, transfer the power, electricity and water bills that may be in their name to their surviving spouse," says estate attorney Doane.

Additionally, Doane notes that some states, such as Florida, require home ownership also be transferred into the name of a living spouse in order for things like title insurance to remain in force.

Since every state has different mandates, be sure to check what type of legal filings, if any, are necessary in the state in which a family member has died, as well as any state where the individual owned property.

Personal Attache
Organizing Financial, Legal and Medical Records

7. Apply for Benefits Due to Survivors

For all kinds of insurance policies, as well as financial contracts -- including car loans, mortgages and credit cards agreements -- find out whether insurance premiums were paid on the accounts. If so, cash benefits may be due to heirs.

Also, ask a lot of questions to find out if survivors are due pension benefits or income from the deceased person's employer, union or maybe even the military. Employers may pay out 401(k) funds, along with unused vacation time, holiday time or bonuses already earned.

For many families, however, the largest lump sum payout following a loved one's death often comes from life insurance proceeds. In dealing with insurers, experts say, the process should be fairly straight-forward.

"You get a claim form and submit it, along with a death certificate," says Canton, the insurance agent. "In most cases, in four to five weeks, you'll get a check."

But Canton warns about the pitfalls of getting a huge life insurance payout -- especially while family members are still grieving. "Sometimes the worst thing you can do is have an insurance company cut (a beneficiary) a check for $500,000," he says, noting that many people blow the money, "just like many lottery winners."

"The best advice I can give people is: Do nothing for six months. Just let the money stay with the insurer, and continue to collect interest," Canton advises.

8. Pay Final Bills and Guard Against Financial Fraud

While paying the final bills for someone who's died, don't forget about things like property taxes or income taxes that may be due. A good CPA can file a final 1040 for the deceased individual and, if required, a Form 1041, an estate income tax return.

Carrying out the duties of an executor also means protecting the deceased person and his or her heirs against financial fraud and exploitation.

There are several ways to do this:

•   Keep the obituary short and sweet. John Sileo, a nationally-known speaker on identity theft and the author of Privacy Means Profit, says, "Share as little information about the person as necessary," because obituaries are easy places for crooks to find a deceased person's age, birth date and sometimes other data like an address or a mother's maiden name Levin puts it bluntly: "The reality is, there are people that case obituaries like burglars case houses."

•   Be careful with social media. It's tempting to go on Facebook or other social networking sites to post tributes, create online memorials and offer personal reflections about a loved one who has died. But experts caution against it. "The more information people give away about their deceased relatives, the more information that identity thieves will be getting," warns Levin, who is also co-founder of Credit.com and Identity Theft 911. Also, don't notify people of someone's death via a social networking site. If you absolutely must use these networks to communicate a death notice, says Sileo, "send a direct message that the person has died and then shut down the account, just like you would financial accounts."

•   Don't toss; shred. If you're cleaning out a loved one's home after their death, be mindful of dumpster divers and others who steal mail. Shred important documents instead of putting them in the trash, Sileo recommends.

•   Limit personal access to sensitive data. Lastly, avoid the mistake of letting copies of the death certificate or personal records lay around unprotected, even in boxes. Take extra care to secure the financial documents of those who had been living in nursing homes or assisted living facilities. "When you're dealing with a chronically-ill person or someone in a nursing home who has died, and the person was often sedated or sleeping, health care workers often have opportunity to rifle through the person's mail and files," Levin notes. "Unfortunately, that can lead to tragic financial events."

Going through all the personal items and economic affairs of someone who has died is bound to be stressful. So do get professional and emotional support if you feel overwhelmed.

And if you're tasked with carrying out what can be a gut-wrenching process, at least let it be a learning experience for you -- and a wake up call to get your own financial house in order.

"You can avoid all sorts of headaches and misery for you and your heirs, and avoid probate and estate taxes too," says Doane, "if you just plan properly before you die."

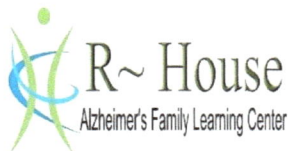

Please contact us if you would like to have a family On-Line Seminar using this guide book.

CONTACT: www.wittsendconsulting@gmail.com

In an effort to further support your family, R~House Alzheimer's Family Learn Center offers an On-Line session for families, we use the www.gotomeeting.com platform.

A member of your family can contact us to set-up a date and time. Our staff will assign links for the members of your family to come up On-Line with a Go-To Meetings webinar for a 45 minute session.

In this session: R~House Alzheimer's Family Learning Center will walk your family through the designed chapters of this study guide to assist you in better application of each section. Together we will address questions that arise from reviewing the book and applying these concepts to your family dynamic.

A reasonable fee will be required prior to set-up the on-line session. Many families choose to do this session from a single site where the families have gathered at one location. In other situations, there have been families with members in several other states, whereby this is a convenient way to bring everyone together for the single purpose of working as a unified family.

You're Not Alone, Take These Seminars

PROVIDED BY: R~House Alzheimer's Family Learning Center

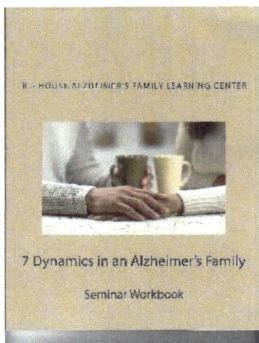

The 7 Dynamics in an Alzheimer's Family, unites the family around the primary caregiver and loved one. There is a lot of work to do as a family. This seminar outlines where to get started. In the seminar the attendee learns how to unite the family, gets an understanding of the disease, how it progresses, learns how to manage dementia related behavior, creates role assignments for family members, is provided templates for creating a proactive plan. 3 Seminars

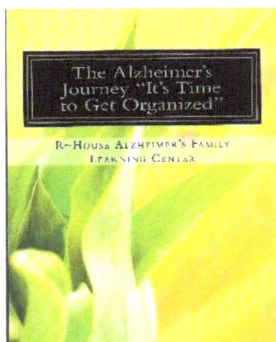

The Alzheimer's Journey, It's Time to get Organized, getting the family organized in the Alzheimer's journey is a matter of taking the right steps. These steps are outlined and reviewed in this seminar. The workbook outlines what to organize, provides templates for setting up organizing binders, planning templates and reference resources. Getting organized reduces stress, save money and gives the family a position of empowerment. 2 Seminars

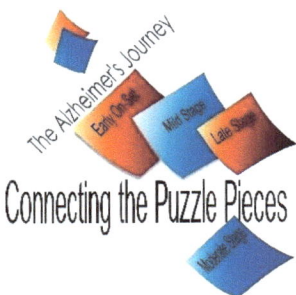

The Alzheimer's Journey, Connecting the Puzzle Pieces, each stage of the disease progression brings about new critical issues, decisions and requirements for proactive planning. The "Connecting the Puzzle Pieces is a five-book series, one for each stage, with a seminar on what to do in each stage. Stages: Early On-Set Stage, Mild Stage, Moderate Stage, Late Stage, End of Life Stage. 1 Seminar

Personal Attache
Organizing Financial, Legal and Medical Records

DISCLOSURE

R~House Alzheimer's Family Learning Center does not provide advise on any and all issues regarding financial, legal or medical. Our focus is to get you educated about Alzheimer's disease and organized for the journey. We strongly recommend that you seek the services of a State Licensed professional before acting on any and all final decisions.

Personal Attache
Organizing Financial, Legal and Medical Records

OUR OTHER PRODUCTS

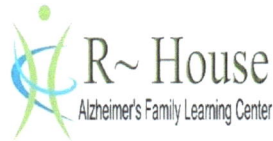

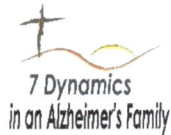

R~ House
Alzheimer's Family Learning Center

FAMILY

7 Dynamics
in an Alzheimer's Family

Educate and Train the <u>Family</u>

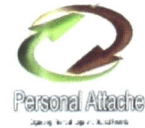

Personal Attache

Organize and Unite the <u>Family</u>

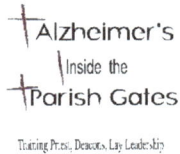

Alzheimer's
Inside the
Parish Gates

Training Priest, Deacons, Lay Leadership

CHURCH

Alzheimer's
Home Reach Ministry

Educate the <u>Church</u> Leaders and Staff

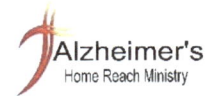

Provide <u>Church</u> Ministry Outreach Model

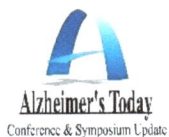

Alzheimer's Today
Conference & Symposium Update

COMMUNITY   **EMPLOYERS**

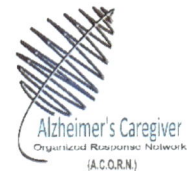

Alzheimer's Caregiver
Organized Response Network
(A.C.O.R.N.)

Bring together the <u>Community</u> Support

A "Wellness Health Plan Benefit" for <u>Employer's</u>

A Complete Response to Support the Alzheimer's Family

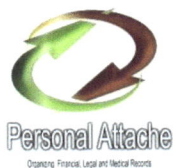

Personal Attache
Organizing Financial, Legal and Medical Records

IN THE END

You are doing all this to support the primary caregiver.

Their decision should carry
the greatest level of decision making authority.

Sirach 3:12-14 Good News Translation (GNT)
12 My child, take care of your father when he grows old; give him no cause for worry as long as he lives. 13 Be sympathetic even if his mind fails him; don't look down on him just because you are strong and healthy. 14 The Lord will not forget the kindness you show to your father; it will help you make up for your sins.

www.ingramcontent.com/pod-product-compliance
Lightning Source LLC
Chambersburg PA
CBHW060808270326
41928CB00002B/28